Medical Marijuana

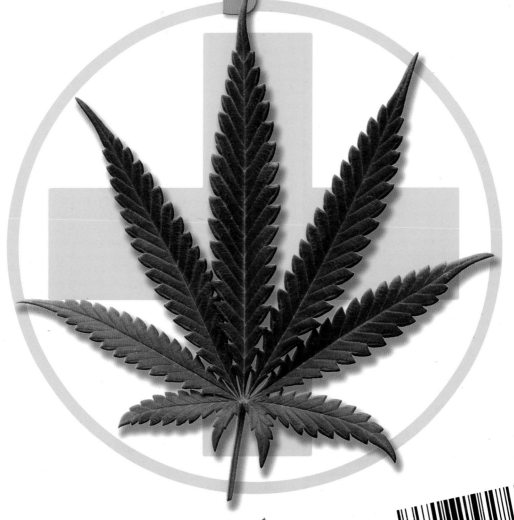

pil

Publications International, Ltd.

D1299721

Written by: Lisa Brooks

Photography: Shutterstock.com and Wikimedia Commons

ISBN: 978-1-64030-587-8

Manufactured in China.

8 7 6 5 4 3 2 1

Table of Contents

Introduction: Changing Perception

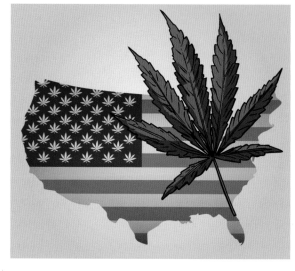

In the 1980s, First Lady Nancy Reagan created the "Just Say No" campaign, which aimed to curb drug use in teens. The simple-but-catchy slogan made its way into popular culture, inspiring "very special episodes" of shows like *Family Ties* and *Diff'rent Strokes*, and sparking a myriad of anti-drug television movies in which stars like Scott Baio, Helen Hunt, and Michelle Pfeiffer demonstrated the dangers of drug use. The "Just Say No" program eventually faded away into the annals of 1980s nostalgia, having shown little evidence of actually being effective. But it paved the way for subsequent campaigns like the "Above the Influence" program and the Drug Abuse Resistance Education—or "D.A.R.E."—program.

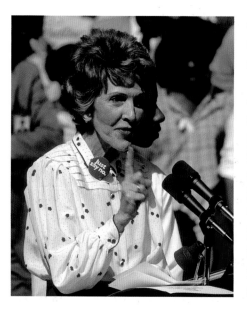

And who can forget the anti-drug commercials? Many of these ads were produced by the non-profit group Partnership for a Drug-Free America (now known as Partnership for Drug-Free Kids). Arguably the most famous commercial featured a man cracking an egg into a hot frying pan and proclaiming, "this is your brain on drugs." Another famous spot showed a father confronting his son with a box of drugs, demanding to know how the boy even knew how to use such shocking items. "I learned it by watching you!" the boy finally admits. More recently, an anti-marijuana commercial aired in which a girl laments the loss of her once fun friend, who has become "lazy and boring" since smoking marijuana.

The effects of the "Just Say No" program are debatable, with some critics saying that the campaign inflamed fears amongst the public, magnified mass incarceration rates, and thwarted youths from receiving accurate information for dealing with drug abuse. The simplistic catchphrase did not address real problems and exacerbated the stigma of drug users as amoral or bad people.

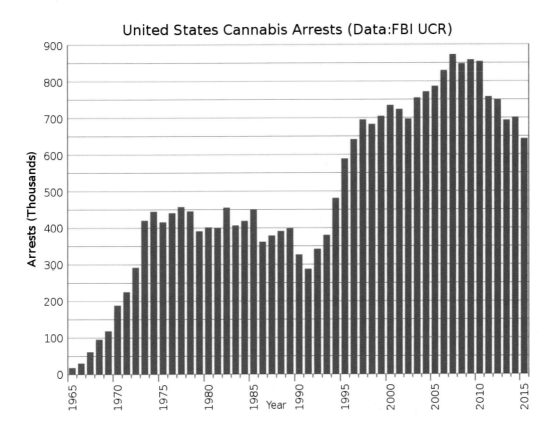

United States Cannabis Arrests (Data:FBI UCR)

A graph depicting the arrest rates for cannabis related offenses in the U.S. from 1965 to 2015.

But in spite of all the slogans, after-school specials, and scare-tactic commercials, marijuana usage has steadily climbed among American adults, with numbers doubling between 2005 and 2015. While teenage use has remained stable over the years, use of the drug continues to rise across all other age groups—from young adults to retirees. This increase in use may be partly due to one simple reason: as of 2018, thirty states have laws which legalize medical or recreational marijuana, and more states consider legalization every year. Proponents of marijuana's use for medical reasons—which include the American College of Physicians, former President Barack Obama, and CNN medical correspondent Dr. Sanjay Gupta—laud the much-maligned drug's many medicinal benefits, giving pause to the validity of all those nostalgic anti-marijuana commercials. Perhaps marijuana—also known as weed, pot, dope, ganja, and literally hundreds of other names—deserves to be seen in a new light.

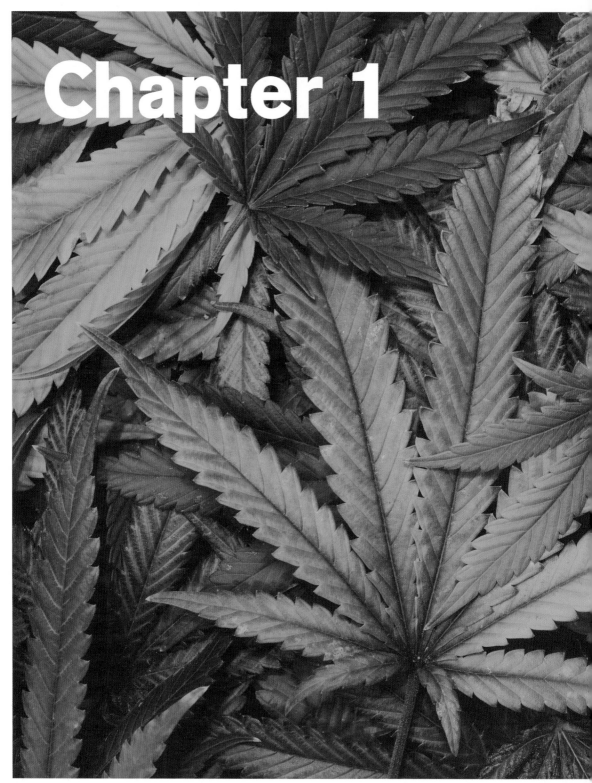

Chapter 1

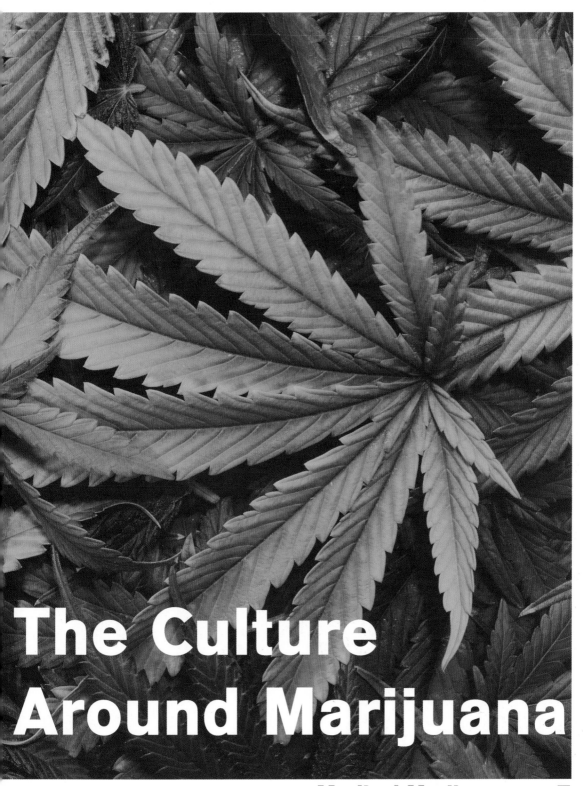

The Culture
Around Marijuana

First, a Little History

Relatively speaking, the United States is very much a newcomer to the marijuana scene. The plant—whose official genus is *Cannabis*—is one of the world's oldest cultivated crops, with its origin going all the way back to the development of agriculture itself. In fact, in 1977, scientist Carl Sagan suggested that cannabis may have been the first cultivated crop in the world. And as many scientists agree that the creation of agriculture was the stepping stone that led to modern civilization, Sagan argues that we may, in fact, have marijuana to thank for human advancement! In his book *The Dragons of Eden: Speculations on the Evolution of Human Intelligence*, Sagan says, "It would be wryly interesting if in human history the cultivation of marijuana led generally to the invention of agriculture, and thereby to civilization." Shines a whole new light on the stereotype of a "stoner," doesn't it?

Ancient Cultivation

Archeologists believe marijuana's use goes back at least 12,000 years. Cannabis probably originated in the area that is now Mongolia, but seeds dating back to 3000 BC have also been found in Siberia and parts of China, and mummified marijuana has been found in the ancient tombs of Chinese nobles. The oldest record of marijuana's medicinal use dates back to 4000 BC, when the plant was used for its anesthetic properties. By 1000 BC, cannabis had made its way to the Middle East and India, where it was prized for its ability to relieve anxiety. It was even mentioned in an ancient sacred Hindu text called *Atharvaveda*—which translates to "Science of Charms"—where it was dubbed "sacred grass."

From South Asia, marijuana's popularity spread to the Greeks and Romans, and its value as a medicinal plant really began to take hold. Roman naturalist Pliny the Elder wrote of its analgesic effects in his book *Naturalis Historia* ("Natural History"); Roman army medic Dioscorides described medical marijuana in his pharmacopoeia, *De Materia Medica* ("On Medical Material"); and famous ancient Greek physician Galen often prescribed marijuana to his patients.

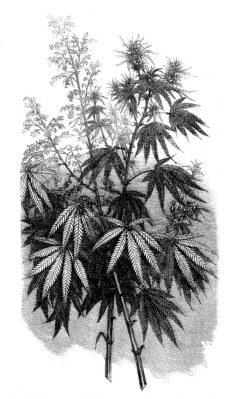

An 1882 engraved illustration of a marijuana plant from the French magazine *La Magasin Pittoresque*.

Cannabis in the New World

Arab traders took the plant south to the Mozambique coast of Africa, and nomadic Indo-European tribes carried the plant further west, where Vikings and Germanic peoples used it as a pain reliever for childbirth and toothaches. For hundreds of years, cannabis remained confined to the world's eastern continents, until the sixteenth century, when Angolan slaves brought plants with them to Brazilian sugar plantations. Over the next several hundred years, marijuana enjoyed increasing popularity within the Americas. By the 1700s, medical marijuana was used in New England, and by the 1800s, the plant was commonly grown on plantations in many southern states, as well as New York and California. Medical marijuana was even easily available for purchase throughout the United States at pharmacies and general stores. After millennia of medical use, it seemed that this versatile drug was poised to become a staple within the medical community. But as anyone can see from the decades-long debate over medical marijuana, things have not been that simple for the cannabis plant.

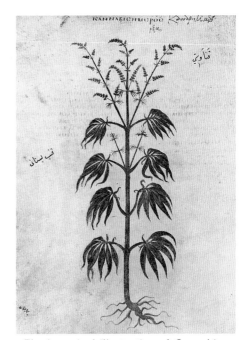

The botanical illustration of *Cannabis sativa* from a Byzantine Greek illuminated manuscript of Dioscorides' *De Materia Medica*. This manuscript was made in 515 AD in Constantinople for the daughter of one of the last Western Roman Emperors, Anicius Olybrius.

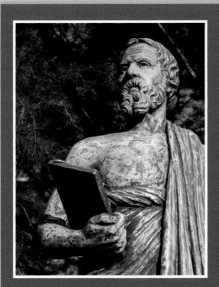

Herodotus' Account of Marijuana Use

Herodotus, the Greek historian who is often considered "The Father of History," gives us one of the earliest records of marijuana use in his 440 BC manuscript, *Histories*. After an encounter with the Scythian people of Eurasia, he recounted their practice of taking baths in cannabis steam. He writes, "The Scythians, as I said, take some of this hemp-seed [presumably flowers], and, creeping under the felt coverings, throw it upon the red-hot stones; immediately it smokes, and gives out such a vapour as no Grecian vapour-bath can exceed; the Scyths, delighted, shout for joy."

Not Just Medicine

There's more than one type of cannabis plant, and the uses of the different types go far beyond medicine. *Cannabis sativa* is the plant that is known for its medicinal and psychoactive properties; but a subspecies, *Cannabis sativa L.*—the "L" in honor of botanist Carl Linnaeus——is more commonly known as hemp. This species of cannabis has little to none of the psychoactive properties of *Cannabis sativa*, making it much more useful for manufacturing products such as cloth and oil.

An Industrious Plant

Hemp's history—like that of its medicinal cousin—goes back thousands of years. It was one of the first plants to be spun into a fiber, and these fibers have been discovered in pottery at archeological sites dating back 10,000 years in what is now Taiwan. Around 6000 BC, the Chinese began using hemp seeds and oil for food, and over the next two thousand years, they learned to weave the fiber into fine textiles. Rope made of hemp was commonly used throughout China, Russia, and Greece by 200 BC. But the Chinese, not content to stop with rope and cloth, next invented hemp paper; eventually, the Arabs learned this technique, as well.

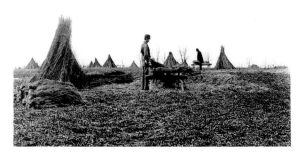

A photo of farmers harvesting hemp in Kentucky. During the nineteenth and twentieth centuries, Kentucky's Bluegrass region was responsible for a majority of the nation's hemp, producing nearly three-fourths of the nation's supply in 1902. According to the Kentucky Historical Society, the first hemp crop was planted in Kentucky in 1775 near Danville, about eighty miles southeast of Louisville.

The journey of hemp's usefulness followed the path of medicinal marijuana, with hemp rope soon showing up in England and other parts of Europe. Hemp cloth became popular, as well, and not just with the common populace: the Merovingian queen Arnegunde was buried with her finest jewelry, and wrapped in a hemp shroud. Over the next several hundred years, hemp rope became standard on European ships—including those used by Christopher Columbus—and the fiber was in high demand. In fact, it was so prized that in 1533 King Henry VIII began fining farmers who refused to grow hemp for industrial use! Spaniards introduced hemp to South America in the mid-sixteenth century, and by the seventeenth century, the Puritans were cultivating the crop in New England. Even the first president of the United States, George Washington, grew hemp and encouraged its cultivation in the new country due to its industrial purposes. The plant became vitally important during World War II, when hemp was used to make uniforms, canvas, and rope. (By the way, if the word *canvas* has a familiar ring to it, that's because it was derived from the word *cannabis*—the material first used to construct it!)

Everything but the High

As our forebears discovered, this amazing plant has a myriad of uses: Hemp seeds are edible and can be used in breads, cereals, or as protein powder. They can even be used to create a vegan "milk." The oil of the seed is useful for ink, paint, cosmetics, and personal care products like lotions and soap. Hemp stalks produce the fibers that have been used for thousands of years to create clothing, paper, shoes, carpets, and rope. More recently, hemp has even been used to create building materials, such as insulating blocks and plaster used in houses, and composite panels used in automobiles.

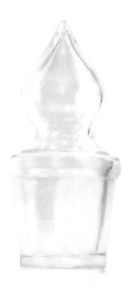

One-hundred milliliters of hemp biodiesel made from hemp seeds, hemp stalks, and alcohol. The inventor of the diesel engine, Rudolph Diesel, originally invented his engine to run on an assortment of fuels, especially vegetable and seed oils.

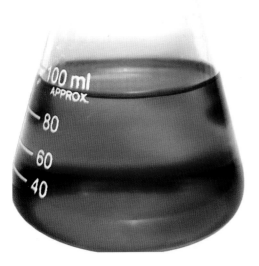

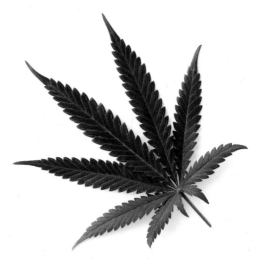

Unfairly Maligned

It would seem that hemp can do just about everything, but there's one thing it can't do: hemp can't give you the "high" associated with *Cannabis sativa*, due to its low concentration of the psychoactive substance tetrahydrocannabinol, or THC. Regardless, the 1937 Marijuana Tax Act began restricting the growth and sale of all forms of cannabis, and in 1970, the Controlled Substances Act categorized both *Cannabis sativa* and *Cannabis sativa L.* as "Schedule I" drugs—despite the fact that hemp lacks any psychoactive properties!

For decades, growing any type of cannabis in the U.S. was illegal—even perfectly innocuous hemp—so most of the hemp used in the country was imported. Because of its prohibition, many people have been unaware of the amazing uses this plant provides and have often equated hemp with its medicinal cousin. But over the last decade, regulations have slowly started to change, and it is now legal to grow hemp in more than a dozen states. Not only that, but more than half of U.S. states have now legalized marijuana for medical use; perhaps hemp is not the only cannabis plant that has been unfairly maligned. On the coming pages, we'll delve into this controversial drug and explore its many promising uses.

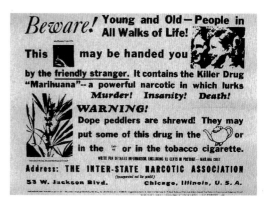

A public service announcement from the Federal Bureau of Narcotics that was used during the 1930s and 1940s to warn the public of the ostensible dangers marijuana then began to pose to the nation's well-being.

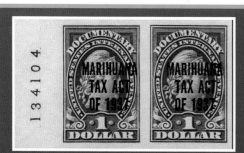

Marihuana Tax Act of 1937

The Marihuana Tax Act of 1937 placed a sales tax on all transactions of cannabis and hemp in the United States until it was repealed in 1969. The act initially gained steam from Harry J. Anslinger of the Federal Bureau of Narcotics in the early 1930s because of his concern of the purported increase of people smoking the plant. Some historians have claimed that the act was passed largely to suppress the hemp industry at the behest of Andrew Mellon, Randolph Hearst, and the Du Pont family, whose investments in timber and nylon were threatened by the cheap alternative that hemp presented.

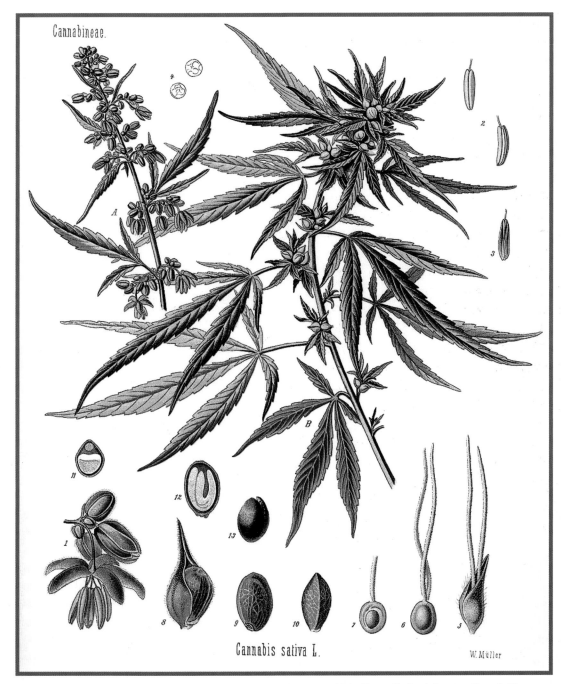

A botanical illustration of the *Cannabis sativa L.* plant. A) Flowering Male Plant, B) Seed-Bearing Female Plant, 1) Male Flower, 2) Pollen Sac, 3) Pollen Sac (different angle), 4) Pollen Grain of Sac, 5) Female Flower With Cover Petal, 6) Female Flower Without Cover Petal, 7) Female Fruit (cross section), 8) Fruit With Cover Petal, 9) Fruit Without Cover Petal, 10) Fruit Without Cover Petal (different angle), 11) Fruit Without Cover Petal (cross section), 12) Fruit Without Cover Petal (longitudinal cross section), 13) Seed Without Hull

A Worldwide Phenomenon

You would think that with its long and notable history—perhaps stretching back to the dawn of agriculture itself—marijuana would be one of the most widely used substances in the world: and you'd be right! Marijuana is the most commonly used drug on the planet, even in countries where it is considered illegal. But many countries around the globe have rather lax laws about the substance, and a few have even legalized it outright. Wondering where to book your next vacation? Here are a few countries to consider:

Uruguay

South America's second-smallest nation is known for its beaches, affordability, and relatively low crime rate compared to the rest of the continent, making it a popular destination for tourists. The country also legalized cannabis for Uruguay nationals in 2013, and it is now legal for citizens to grow, buy, sell, and consume the plant. Uruguay also recently became the first country in the world to sell marijuana in pharmacies. The only catch is that citizens and pharmacies must register with the government if they plan to partake. But again, this only applies to Uruguay nationals.

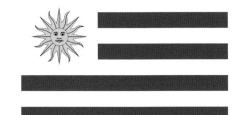

Portugal

In 2001, Portugal made headlines when it decriminalized drugs—and not just cannabis, but "harder" drugs like cocaine and heroin, as well. The country implemented a policy based on treatment plans for those who are addicted to drugs, as opposed to punitive penalties, and as a result has seen a decline in heroin and cocaine addiction. Possession of cannabis for personal use was also decriminalized, but ironically it is still illegal to cultivate the plant, even for personal use. As a result, most Portuguese cannabis users illegally acquire the substance from Spain, even though possessing it cannot lead to criminal charges. It's an interesting juxtaposition between legal and illegal; but many agree that Portugal's drug policy is a step in the right direction and that other countries—including the United States—should definitely take notice.

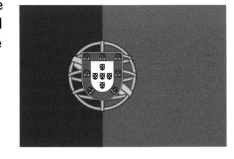

Switzerland

Switzerland is famous for several things: delicious chocolate, well-made watches, and private banking, to name a few. They're also notoriously neutral when it comes to world conflict; but in the case of cannabis, the Swiss have taken a side. The country has decriminalized the possession of marijuana for personal use, and has made cannabis with less than one percent THC perfectly legal. This THC amount isn't enough to give users a "high," but it's still said to be effective for relieving pain and anxiety. Switzerland was also the first country to sell hemp cigarettes in supermarkets, which have proven to be extremely popular.

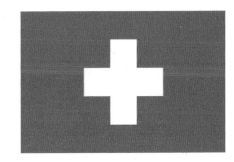

Netherlands

Everyone has heard stories about the famous coffee houses in Amsterdam, the largest city in the Netherlands. With more than 250 of these marijuana-friendly establishments in the city, residents and tourists can explore different varieties and strains of their favorite recreational drug, right alongside a cup of cappuccino or a pastry. What's unusual is that technically, marijuana is illegal in the country; but it's so pervasive that authorities usually look the other way. Paradoxically, Amsterdam's cannabis coffee houses are totally legal, each one possessing a permit to conduct business. For tourists, this means that cannabis consumption is mostly limited to Amsterdam's coffee houses.

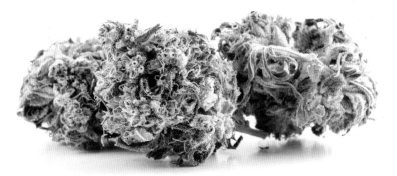

Canada

Our neighbor to the north legalized marijuana for medical use back in 2001. Today, Prime Minister Justin Trudeau—who has admitted to smoking marijuana himself—has been working to legalize cannabis for recreational use throughout the entire country. And his campaign has worked: at the end of 2017, the Canadian House of Commons voted overwhelmingly in favor of legalization, 200 votes to 82. This means that soon, Americans will be able to hop over the border and legally buy and consume the drug, perhaps hanging out in Amsterdam-style coffee houses in downtown Toronto.

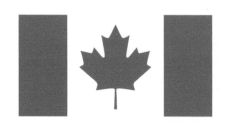

Other Countries

Other cannabis-friendly countries include Peru, Jamaica, Ecuador, and Costa Rica, which allow adults to possess small amounts of marijuana for personal use. Medical marijuana is legal for limited instances in Italy and Australia. And in Argentina, marijuana is not only legal for medical use, but it's free for individuals who qualify. But if traveling abroad seems like a drastic measure to buy some cannabis, take heart: policies are constantly changing right here in America, with more and more states embracing the idea of marijuana legalization.

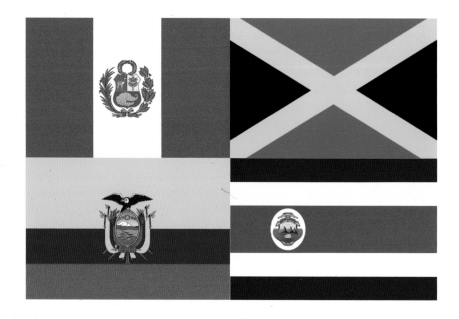

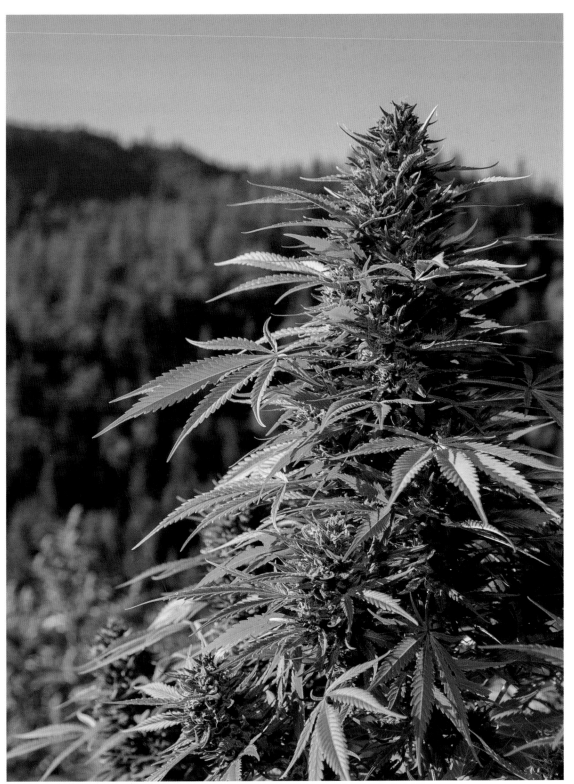

It All Began in Mexico

It seems that marijuana's journey is coming full circle. For millennia it was freely used by cultures around the world, even in the United States. But as the anti-drug campaigns of the late twentieth century demonstrated, the drug fell out of favor and was considered illegal for decades; today, however, marijuana is rebounding. The many benefits of the plant are starting to draw the attention of even the most straightlaced teetotalers, and little by little, the drug is regaining legal ground.

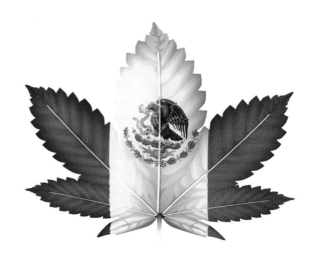

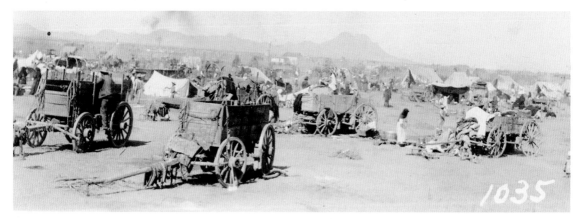

A photo, circa 1914, of refugees fleeing the violence of the Mexican Revolution.

Border-Crossing Customs

But why was this time-tested, widely used plant ever criminalized to begin with? The answer dates back to 1910, when the Mexican Revolution caused great unrest in the country. Mexican immigrants began fleeing to states like Texas and Louisiana to escape the violence, and the newcomers, of course, brought their customs and culture with them. One of the customs they enjoyed was the use of marijuana as a recreational drug. Americans were used to the substance as medicine; cannabis was widely available in pharmacies across the country. But this new, recreational use of marijuana was a novel idea. In fact, even the word *marijuana* was foreign to Americans, as the word *cannabis* was always used for the popular tinctures and medicines in pharmacies.

The Spanish-speaking immigrants who arrived in the country were often met with prejudice and suspicion. And these attitudes were also expressed towards their custom of marijuana use. The media caught on to the public's distrust of Mexican immigrants, and began to rail against the foreigners, painting a picture of violent and disruptive immigrants and raising fears in Americans. Authorities began to blame the "violence" of these immigrants on their use of marijuana, calling it a "killer weed" that gave its users "superhuman strength," and warning the public that Mexicans were handing out the drug to innocent schoolchildren. Americans, unaware that this "marijuana" was the very same cannabis that sat in their medicine cabinets, were convinced that the immigrants had introduced a dangerous new drug to the country.

National Paranoia

By 1931, twenty-nine states had outlawed marijuana, even though there was no evidence that the drug was particularly dangerous. But the public's perception of the drug—fueled by fear and prejudice against the Mexican immigrants—along with propaganda like the 1936 film *Reefer Madness*, eventually led to the Marijuana Tax Act of 1937, which enacted country-wide penalties for anyone who bought or sold cannabis. And in the 1950s, federal laws were created that made the penalties even stricter: a first offense conviction for possession of marijuana could carry a sentence of two to ten years in prison and a $20,000 fine!

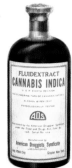

Cannabis indica has been used for recreational and medicinal applications more often than *Cannabis sativa* because of its higher levels of THC and CBD.

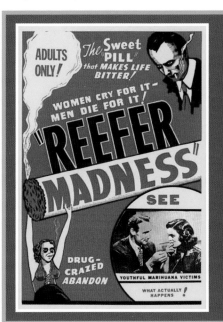

Reefer Madness

Reefer Madness is a propaganda film that follows the downfall of a group of high-school students who become addicted to marijuana. In the film, the students commit multiple crimes, including a hit and run accident, manslaughter, and rape, and also suffer from hallucinations because of their use of marijuana. Although it was originally conceived as a moral tale to inform parents of the dangers of marijuana, it was later bought by producer Dwain Esper to be re-cut as an exploitation film. Many decades later, the film was rediscovered and became a cult classic as an unintentional satire.

Unfair Stigma

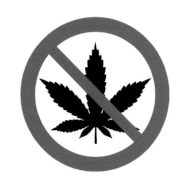

After thousands of years of use around the world, suddenly cannabis was reduced from hero to villain in mere decades. And just as quickly, marijuana developed a reputation—and certainly not a good one. More and more people were using the drug for recreational purposes as opposed to medicinally, and many Americans felt that "getting high" wasn't a good enough reason to consume cannabis. Instead of being seen as a medicinal marvel with a relatively safe track record, the drug was now considered a dangerous substance only used by drug addicts. This was despite the fact that the medicines Americans had been using for decades and the "new" drug marijuana were one and the same!

Skewed Cultural Perception

Before its criminalization, marijuana was often described in a way that would spread fear amongst the public, with authorities insisting that its use led to violence and even insanity. These perceptions didn't last long, since the effects of marijuana are often completely opposite—in fact, many people use the drug to unwind, relax, and quell anxiety.

But this led to another stigma: the idea that cannabis users are lazy, unmotivated, and unproductive members of society. Consider the anti-marijuana commercial with the "lazy and boring" girl on the couch: this stereotype became pervasive in the United States, causing anyone who didn't want to be seen as "lazy and boring" to shamefully hide their marijuana use. But with around 55 million regular marijuana users in the U.S., chances are we all know someone who uses the drug now and then—they probably just don't want to admit it!

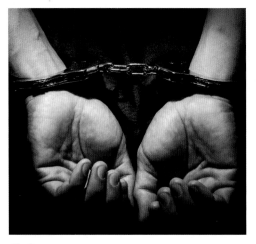

A tremendous amount of resources are used toward battling drug use in the U.S., with one quarter of all prisoners being detained for drug related crimes. Although our government has spent trillions of dollars over the last forty years to battle drug use, the rates of drug use have not decreased. The ACLU reports that fifty-two percent of all drug arrests in 2010 were for marijuana, and out of the eight million marijuana arrests made between 2001 and 2010, eighty-eight percent of those arrests were simply for possessing it. The ACLU also reports that despite relatively equal rates of consumption of marijuana between white and black populations, black populations are nearly four times more likely to be arrested for marijuana.

Left Out of the Conversation

Perhaps the worst consequence of the stereotypes and stigmas surrounding cannabis is that they have prevented many from seeing the drug as a viable medicinal remedy. Even with thousands of years of use and evidence to back up the claim of marijuana's medicinal prowess, efforts to legalize the plant have been slow going. Some scoff at the idea that the drug is good for anything other than a "high," while others are interested in trying the remedy, but worry about the social stigma that might follow. And that's too bad, because cannabis has shown plenty of promising results when used for a host of ailments.

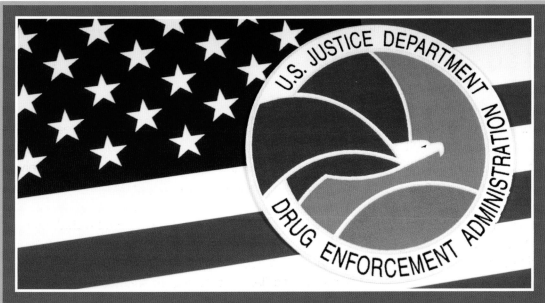

Classified by the DEA

Marijuana is federally classified as a Schedule I Controlled Substance, meaning that the federal government believes marijuana has a high potential for abuse and the potential to cause severe psychological and physical dependence. Schedule I drugs have no currently accepted medical use. Marijuana is currently a Schedule I drug along with heroin, LSD, ecstasy, Quaaludes, and peyote. The DEA identifies the effects of marijuana as:

- Dizziness, facial flushing, dry mouth
- Happiness, exhilaration at high doses
- Disinhibition, relaxation, increased sociability, talkativeness
- Enhanced sensory perception, increased appreciation of art and music
- Increase in imagination and perceived creativity
- Distortion of time
- Illusions, delusions
- Increased appetite
- Emotional lability, dysphoria, confusion, restlessness, anxiety

An Ineffective War

In 1970, President Richard Nixon signed the Controlled Substances Act into law, which established a federal drug policy. Recreational drug use had steadily climbed throughout the 1960s, and by the end of the decade nearly half of Americans believed that drug abuse was a serious problem in the country. Nixon proclaimed it "public enemy number one," and by June 1971 the president had officially declared a "War on Drugs."

As part of his strategy, Nixon increased federal funding for drug-control agencies and enacted strict penalties for drug offenses, including fines and mandatory prison time. In 1973, Nixon created the Drug Enforcement Administration (DEA), which consisted of 1,470 agents running on a budget of $75 million.

Just Say No

After Nixon left office, the War on Drugs calmed down a bit, with eleven states even passing laws to decriminalize marijuana. But in the 1980s, the conflict began anew, with Nancy Reagan's "Just Say No" campaign and a refocus on penalizing nonviolent drug crime. People began criticizing drug laws, with some believing they unfairly targeted people of color.

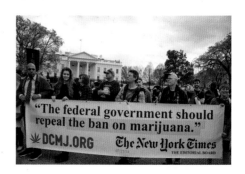

Interestingly, in the early 1980s less than six percent of Americans felt that drug abuse was a major issue in the country; but by the end of the decade—after years of hearing the "Just Say No" slogan—that number had climbed to sixty-four percent. Is it possible that an anti-drug campaign actually caused anti-drug hysteria?

Protesters rally for the legalization of marijuana on April 2, 2016, outside of the White House.

Although anti-drug sentiment began declining by the 1990s, the stigma surrounding marijuana use remained. President Bill Clinton once famously said that he tried marijuana in his younger days, but "didn't inhale." There may have been few people who actually believed his claim, but whether true or not, it's easy to understand why the leader of the country would deny using the substance. But a couple decades later, President Barack Obama had a different answer when asked about his drug use: "When I was a kid, I inhaled frequently. That was the point," he said. Obama's candid statement echoed the changing attitudes toward cannabis in the twenty-first century—attitudes that have led to more and more states jumping on the legalization bandwagon.

Excessive Mass Incarceration

And yet, more than 700,000 people are still arrested for marijuana offenses every year. Decades after its inception, the DEA now employs 5,000 agents and has a budget that exceeds an astounding $2 billion. But after so much money has been spent and so many people arrested, Americans still frequently use marijuana. In fact, in 1969, just before the War on Drugs began, only four percent of Americans had experimented with the drug. But today, that number stands at thirty-eight percent. Clearly, the expensive "War on Drugs" has been a failure.

Perceived Risk of Marijuana Use

A 2016 report on data collected between 2012 and 2014 shows that there are great regional differences in perceived risk of monthly marijuana use. The study concludes that an annual average of nearly 75 million people in the U.S. believe that there is a large risk of harm from monthly marijuana smoking. That averages to about two out of every seven people, or about twenty-eight percent of the population in the U.S. These perceptions are largely held in the South, with sixteen of the highest percentage areas being found in the region. The sixteen lowest percentage areas were found along the Eastern Seaboard and the West Coast.

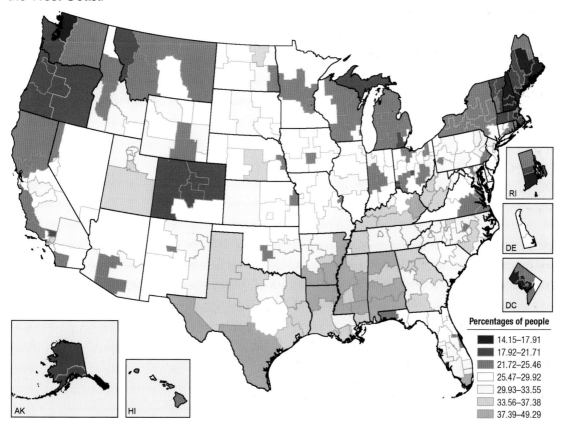

Percentages of people

- 14.15–17.91
- 17.92–21.71
- 21.72–25.46
- 25.47–29.92
- 29.93–33.55
- 33.56–37.38
- 37.39–49.29

A Few Holdouts

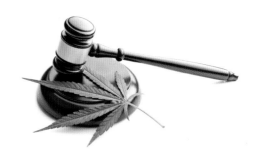

In a moment, we'll talk about the thirty states that have medicinal or recreational laws that legalize marijuana in some form. Another sixteen states have legalized medicinal cannabis with low THC amounts or for patients with specific conditions.

But four states have no laws on the books that legalize marijuana in any form: Idaho, Kansas, Nebraska, and South Dakota. In these states, getting caught with even a small amount of cannabis could result in a hefty penalty.

Idaho

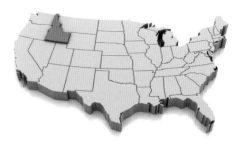

In Idaho, possessing less than three ounces of marijuana is considered a misdemeanor, but it's still punishable by up to one year in prison and a $1,000 fine. More than three ounces? That can get you five years in prison and a $10,000 fine. And it doesn't look like Idaho is planning to change their outlook anytime soon: in 2013, the Idaho legislature approved a statement which reiterated their belief that cannabis should never be legalized. So far, the plant's future in Idaho looks bleak.

Kansas

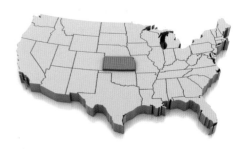

Kansas has shown a bit more progress in the marijuana matter, with efforts being put forth to legalize the plant for medicinal purposes. Wichita, the largest city in the state, also voted to decriminalize the drug, reducing the penalty for first-time possession from a $2,500 fine to just $50. But in the rest of the state, a first-time charge can result not only in the fine, but a year in prison, as well. And subsequent offenses are even harsher, with fines up to $100,000 and three and a half years in prison.

Nebraska

Nebraska has taken a small step towards legalization by decriminalizing a first offense for marijuana possession. Offenders may be fined up to $300 and asked to attend drug education classes, but prison time isn't required. The state is less lenient on repeat offenders, as well, with second or third offenses resulting in a $500 fine and up to a week in jail. Interestingly, marijuana grows wild in Nebraska, where it is known as "ditch weed" and contains very low levels of THC, but millions of these possibly beneficial plants are destroyed each year.

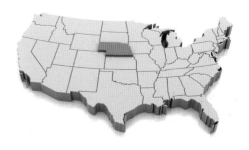

South Dakota

South Dakota is another state that has made attempts to legalize medicinal marijuana, but so far without success. But in November 2017, activists were able to collect enough signatures on a petition to introduce medical cannabis on the 2018 ballot, so there's still hope that something may soon change. In the meantime, possession of a small amount of the drug can result in a $2,000 fine and a year in prison.

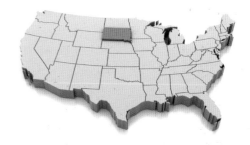

Even though there are still a few holdouts in the march toward country-wide legalization (we're looking at you, Idaho!), the shifting attitude in the United States towards cannabis is obviously starting to make serious strides towards an acceptance of the drug.

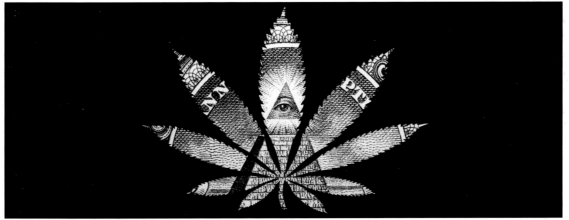

Federal vs. State

Every year, more states vote to legalize marijuana, either for recreational or medicinal use. This is great news for proponents of the drug, but there's one caveat: federally, the drug remains illegal. This means that even if you are following state law when you buy or consume marijuana, you are still breaking federal law. Technically, you could even be charged with a federal crime. And federal law enforcement could potentially shut down cannabis-based businesses in states where such businesses are legal.

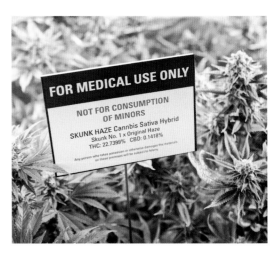

Federal Hurdles and Roadblocks

This disconnect between state and federal laws has other ramifications, as well. For instance, many businesses that sell marijuana are cash-only establishments, because banks are wary about working with businesses that are breaking federal law. And a nervous bank is unlikely to make a loan to such a business. Cannabis-based businesses also can't file for certain tax deductions, thanks to section 280E of the federal tax code, which was originally aimed at illegal drug dealers. This means that a marijuana business can't deduct expenses like advertising, transportation, or rent, resulting in outlandish income tax rates that can exceed ninety percent. These roadblocks add up to a very expensive endeavor—obviously much more than a conventional business.

And those aren't the only hurdles faced by state-legal marijuana establishments. For instance, federal laws prohibit federally controlled water from being used for illegal marijuana farms—and since the drug is still illegal as far as the federal government is concerned, that includes farms in states where marijuana has been legalized. Marijuana farmers work around this by drilling wells or tapping into a city's water supply, but it's just one more inconvenience they must endure in order to run their business.

Because of the threat of a federal-government crackdown in states where marijuana is now medicinally and recreationally available, doctors may not prescribe medical marijuana without violating federal law and risking prosecution or losing their license. They may, however, recommend the therapy to a patient, but it's up to the patient to proceed from there.

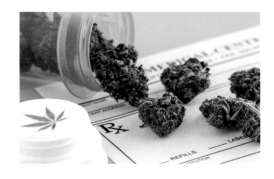

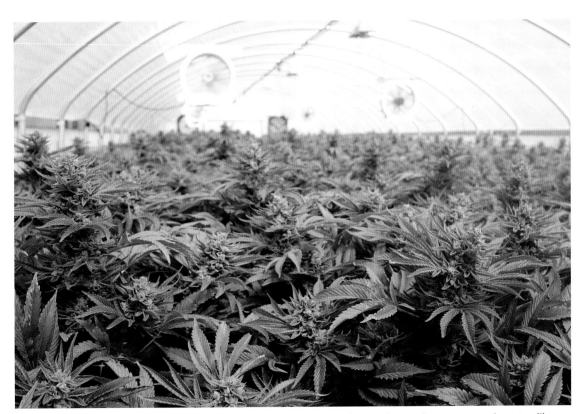

It can be a hassle and an economic burden to find a reliable source of water for marijuana growers in states like California and Colorado because of the federal government's restrictions. But thankfully, marijuana requires much less water to grow than many other crops we grow today. You can grow a marijuana plant with a two-pound bud yield with 480 gallons of water. That may sound like a lot, but producing a pound of beef is said to need 1,500 gallons of water. Almost as bad, it takes one gallon of water to grow a single almond, or 1,000 gallons of water for a can of almonds.

Perhaps worst of all, the DEA is allowed to conduct raids on marijuana establishments, even in states where the drug is legal and the proprietors follow all state laws. Occasionally these raids are justifiable: there have been cases where owners of cannabis-based businesses have participated in money laundering or have even partnered with drug cartels. Others may have state-legal businesses but grow marijuana to illegally ship over the border into states where the drug is still illegal. But many DEA raids hit businesses that comply with all state laws, adding one more worry to the list of complications that owners of marijuana enterprises face.

Federal laws can also pose a problem for those who aren't engaged in selling the drug, but simply wish to use marijuana now and then, whether for recreation or for medical reasons. Since marijuana is still federally illegal, employers in any state—even those with legalization laws—can prohibit use of the drug as a condition of employment. The same holds true for renters: landlords can prohibit residents from using the substance, even in states where it is legal.

One Through Five

When the Controlled Substances Act was signed into law back in 1970, it established five different classifications—called "Schedules"—to help lawmakers and the medical industry decide how best to handle specific drugs. According to the DEA, drugs are assigned a Schedule "depending upon the drug's acceptable medical use and the drug's abuse or dependency potential." Drugs that are considered Schedule I are said to have a high risk for abuse and low potential for medicinal value; conversely, Schedule V drugs have a low risk for abuse and are commonly used as medicine.

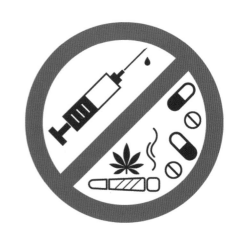

Low Abuse, Medicinal Use

Schedule V drugs may contain low amounts of narcotics, but the potential for abusing these drugs is generally the lowest of all the Schedules. The drugs contained in this classification include antidiarrheal substances like Lomotil, Motofen, and Parepectolin, the pain reliever Lyrica, and cough suppressants with codeine, such as Robitussin AC.

Schedule IV drugs have more of an abuse risk but are commonly used for medical reasons. These include sedatives like Valium, Ambien, and Ativan, the antianxiety medication Xanax, analgesics like Darvocet and Tramadol, and certain muscle relaxers.

Next up are the Schedule III drugs, which include substances with less than ninety milligrams of codeine per dose, such as Tylenol with codeine. Some others in this Schedule are anabolic steroids, testosterone, and the anesthetic Ketamine. As we go higher on the Schedule scale, the drugs ostensibly become more dangerous.

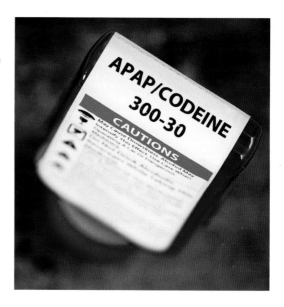

Although codeine isn't considered as dangerous as many other controlled substances, there are several side effects that can be cause for concern. Like all opioid-based pain killers, there is a risk of developing a physical dependence to the drug after prolonged use. This may cause an extreme craving for the drug, nausea, vomiting, chills, irritability, weakness, and insomnia.

High Abuse, Medically Obtuse

Schedule II drugs have a high risk for abuse and potential for physical and psychological addiction. Drugs in this classification include some commonly abused substances like cocaine, methamphetamine, and oxycodone, as well as pain relievers like Vicodin, Demerol, and fentanyl, and stimulants used to treat attention deficit/hyperactivity disorder such as Adderall and Ritalin.

At the very top of the list are the Schedule I drugs, which are not only considered to have a high risk of dependence, but also are believed to have no medicinal use. The drugs in this category include heroin, lysergic acid diethylamide (commonly known as LSD), ecstasy, peyote, and so-called "magic" mushrooms.

Oh, and there's one more drug that joins the Schedule I list: Marijuana.

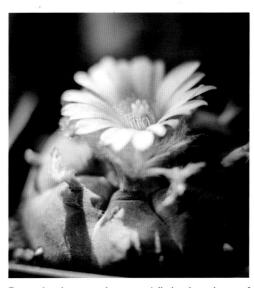

Peyote has been used ceremonially by the cultures of Mexico and the American Southwest for thousands of years for healing and religious practices. But today, its effects are considered malicious enough to be classified as a Schedule I substance.

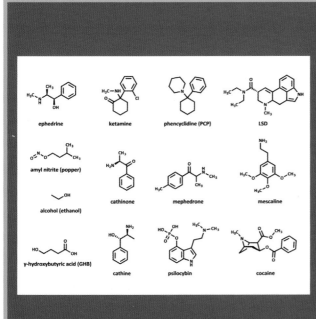

ephedrine   ketamine   phencyclidine (PCP)   LSD

amyl nitrite (popper)

alcohol (ethanol)   cathinone   mephedrone   mescaline

γ-hydroxybutyric acid (GHB)   cathine   psilocybin   cocaine

Scheduled Molecules

Ephedrine is not a controlled substance but it is on List I of over-the-counter substances that can be used to make a controlled substance. Ketamine is a Schedule III anesthetic. PCP is a Schedule II substance that was originally used as an anesthetic. LSD is a Schedule I psychedelic. Poppers are not a scheduled substance. Alcohol is an unscheduled over-the-counter psychoactive sedative. Cathinone is a Schedule I stimulant. Mephedrone is a Schedule I synthetic stimulant. Mescaline is a Schedule I psychedelic. GHB is a Schedule I psychoactive. Cathine is a Schedule IV stimulant. Psilocybin is a Schedule I psychedelic found in mushrooms. Cocaine is a Schedule II stimulant.

A Catch 22

If you think it seems like a bit of overkill to place marijuana in the same category as heroin and LSD (and to place it in a higher category than cocaine and methamphetamine!) you're definitely not alone. After all, drugs like heroin, fentanyl, and oxycodone result in the deaths of approximately 115 Americans every day due to fatal overdoses. And the numbers are rising at a frightening pace: between 2015 and 2016, deaths due to opioid overdoses rose an astounding twenty-eight percent.

Ever-Present Dangers

Drugs that are lower on the Schedule list have risks, as well. For example, acetaminophen, the main ingredient in the Schedule III drug Tylenol with codeine, sends thousands of people to the hospital every year, and can result in fatal liver toxicity. Even substances that seem innocuous, like the Schedule V cough suppressants, can be misused and have been known to cause illness and death.

So why is marijuana, which has a much safer track record than heroin, cocaine, and even acetaminophen, included in the top category of the drug Schedule? The answer has less to do with any "danger" associated with cannabis and more to do with its medical potential—or, as far as the DEA is concerned, lack thereof. Drugs included in Schedule I are considered to have no medicinal benefit. They are believed to be useless for therapeutic use; but every other category, from Schedule II to Schedule V, includes drugs that are used, at least occasionally, for medical purpose. Yes, even cocaine—which can be used as a topical anesthetic—and methamphetamine—which can be used to treat ADHD or as a weight-loss drug—are considered more medically beneficial than marijuana! And it's interesting to note that two widely used (and abused) drugs with no medicinal benefit—alcohol and tobacco—were given special exemptions from the Schedule list. Otherwise, they would certainly fall into the Schedule I category.

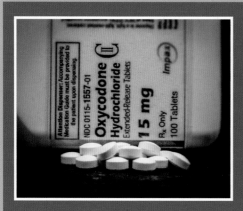

The Opioid Epidemic

Oxycodone is the most popular recreationally used opioid in the U.S., with 11 million people in the U.S. using the drug recreationally annually. But despite their popularity, opioids, synthetic and natural, are extremely dangerous. The opioid epidemic has hit the newsstands as deaths related to opioid abuse have spiked in recent years. According to the National Institute of Drug Abuse, nearly 64,000 people died from opioid overdoses in 2016.

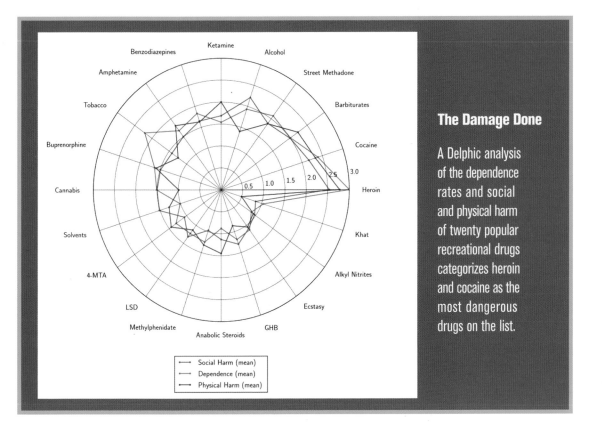

The Damage Done

A Delphic analysis of the dependence rates and social and physical harm of twenty popular recreational drugs categorizes heroin and cocaine as the most dangerous drugs on the list.

Insufficient Proof

The only reason cannabis remains a Schedule I drug is because there is insufficient scientific proof of its medical benefit. With thousands of years of anecdotal evidence and modern users who swear by its effectiveness, you would think that cannabis would at least be given a chance to prove itself.

But herein lies the problem: in order for marijuana to be rescheduled, it needs to be scientifically studied in controlled environments on a large scale, to collect enough evidence to prove its medical worth. But in order to conduct studies, researchers must get the approval of the DEA, which restricts how much marijuana can be researched. The very agency which requires scientific proof to reschedule a drug is restricting the study of that drug—so poor cannabis remains stuck at Schedule I.

But there is hope: the federal government has recently started easing some of the restrictions against studying marijuana, allowing researchers more access to the plant and enabling them to conduct larger studies. This could provide the proof of medicinal benefit needed to move the drug from Schedule I to Schedule II, although it wouldn't necessarily guarantee legal access for all.

Medicinal States

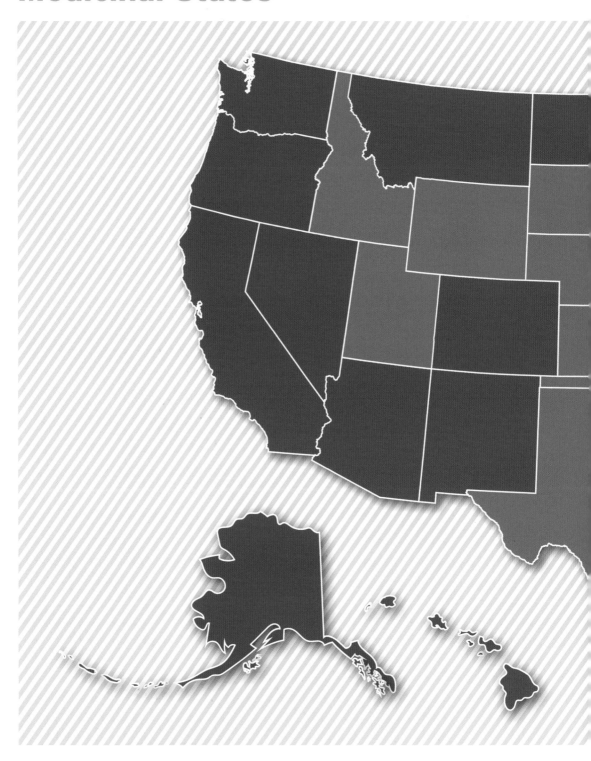

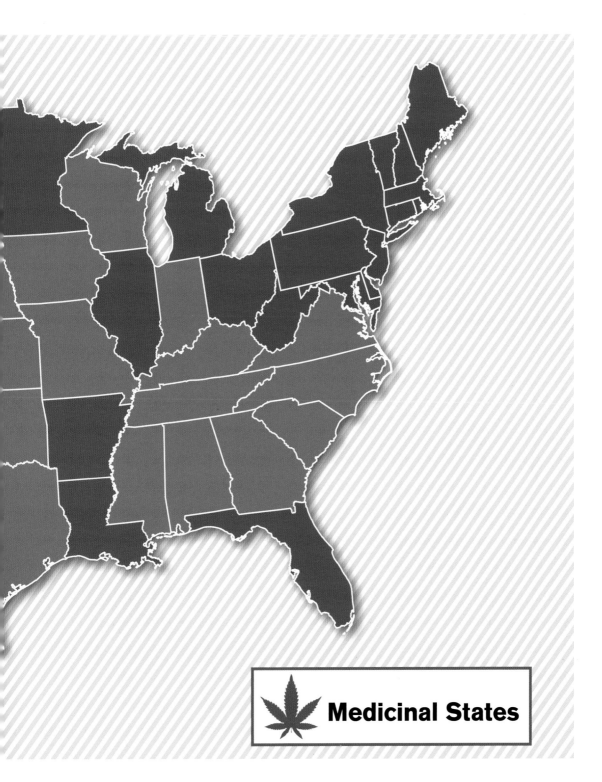

Medicinal States

As of 2018, thirty states and the District of Columbia have laws that make medical marijuana legal. These states include Alaska, Arizona, Arkansas, California, Colorado, Connecticut, Delaware, Florida, Hawaii, Illinois, Louisiana, Maine, Maryland, Massachusetts, Michigan, Minnesota, Montana, Nevada, New Hampshire, New Jersey, New Mexico, New York, North Dakota, Ohio, Oregon, Pennsylvania, Rhode Island, Vermont, Washington, and West Virginia. All of these states require proof of residency to acquire cannabis, to prevent out-of-state visitors from taking advantage of the system.

Each state also provides medical marijuana only for certain medical conditions (sorry, no marijuana for the common cold!), and several states do not allow the drug to be smoked. The following is a state-by-state look at which medical conditions are covered under medicinal marijuana laws:

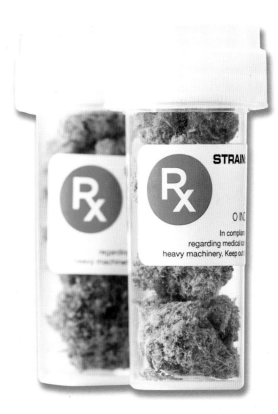

Alaska

Alaska's law covers cancer, glaucoma, HIV or AIDS, or any chronic or debilitating disease or treatment for such diseases, which produces conditions that may be alleviated by the medical use of marijuana: weakness; severe pain; severe nausea; seizures, including those that are characteristic of epilepsy; or persistent muscle spasms, including those that are characteristic of multiple sclerosis. Other conditions are subject to approval by the Alaska Department of Health and Social Services.

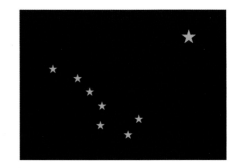

Arizona

Cancer, glaucoma, HIV/AIDS, Hepatitis C, Amyotrophic lateral sclerosis (also known as ALS or Lou Gehrig's disease), Crohn's disease, Alzheimer's disease, wasting syndrome, severe and chronic pain, severe nausea, seizures (including epilepsy), severe or persistent muscle spasms (including multiple sclerosis), and post traumatic stress disorder (PTSD) are all covered.

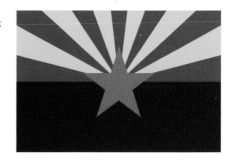

Arkansas

In Arkansas, cannabis can be used for cancer, glaucoma, HIV/AIDS, hepatitis C, ALS, Tourette syndrome, Crohn's disease, ulcerative colitis, PTSD, severe arthritis, fibromyalgia, and Alzheimer's disease. The law also allows its use for any chronic or debilitating disease or medical condition or its treatment that produces one or more of the following: wasting syndrome; peripheral neuropathy; pain that has not responded to ordinary medications, treatment, or surgical measures for more than six months; severe nausea; seizures, including without limitation those characteristic of epilepsy; or severe and persistent muscle spasms, including without limitation those characteristic of multiple sclerosis. Any other medical condition or its treatment must be approved by the Arkansas Department of Health.

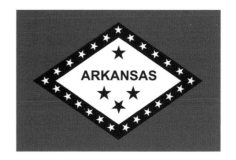

California

AIDS, anorexia, arthritis, wasting syndrome, cancer, chronic pain, glaucoma, migraine, persistent muscle spasms (including spasms associated with multiple sclerosis), seizures (including seizures associated with epilepsy), and severe nausea are covered, as well as other chronic or persistent medical conditions.

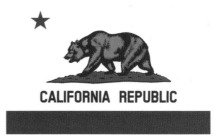

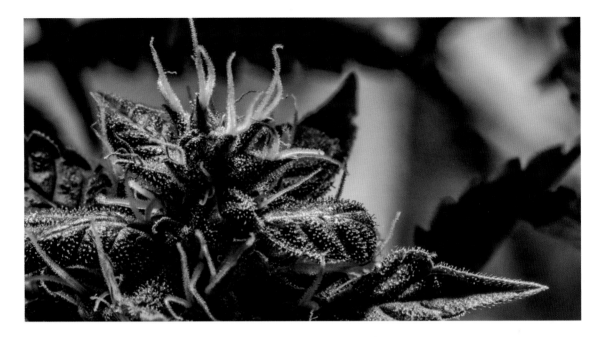

Colorado

Colorado's marijuana laws cover cancer, glaucoma, HIV/AIDS, wasting syndrome, severe pain or severe nausea, seizures (including those that are characteristic of epilepsy), persistent muscle spasms (including those that are characteristic of multiple sclerosis), and PTSD. Other conditions are subject to approval by the Colorado Board of Health.

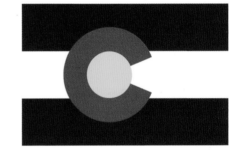

Connecticut

Adults in the state may use cannabis for cancer, glaucoma, HIV/AIDS, Parkinson's Disease, multiple sclerosis, damage to the nervous tissue of the spinal cord with muscle spasticity, epilepsy, wasting syndrome, Crohn's Disease, PTSD, sickle cell disease, chronic pain, severe psoriasis and psoriatic arthritis, ALS, ulcerative colitis, cerebral palsy, cystic fibrosis, terminal illness requiring end-of-life care, and uncontrolled intractable seizure disorder Patients under the age of eighteen may use the drug for cerebral palsy, cystic fibrosis, irreversible spinal cord injuries, severe epilepsy, terminal illness requiring end-of-life care, and uncontrolled intractable seizure disorder.

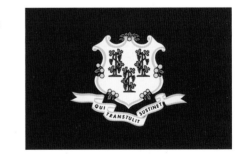

Delaware

For adults, the drug many be used for terminal illness, cancer, HIV/AIDS, severe liver cirrhosis, ALS, Alzheimer's disease, PTSD, epilepsy, multiple sclerosis, and autism with self-injurious or aggressive behavior. Cannabis may also be used for chronic or debilitating diseases or medical conditions or treatments that produce wasting syndrome, severe, debilitating pain that does not respond to prescribed medication or surgical measures, or serious side effects such as intractable nausea, seizures, or severe and persistent muscle spasms.

Patients under the age of eighteen may use cannabis for epilepsy, or any chronic or debilitating disease or medical condition which has caused wasting syndrome, intractable nausea, or severe, painful, and persistent muscle spasms.

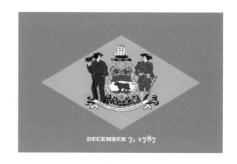

Florida

Cancer, epilepsy, glaucoma, HIV/AIDS, PTSD, ALS, Crohn's disease, Parkinson's disease, multiple sclerosis, chronic pain, and terminal conditions are all covered under Florida's laws.

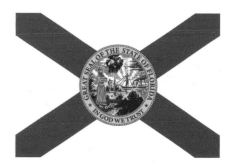

Hawaii

Hawaii's laws cover cancer, glaucoma, HIV/AIDS, and PTSD, as well as chronic or debilitating diseases or medical conditions or treatments that produce wasting syndrome, severe pain, severe nausea, seizures (including those characteristic of epilepsy), or severe and persistent muscle spasms (including those characteristic of multiple sclerosis or Crohn's disease). Any other conditions are subject to approval by the Hawaii Department of Health.

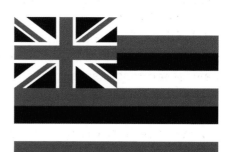

Illinois

In Illinois, cannabis may be used for ailments including Alzheimer's disease, HIV/AIDS, ALS, Arnold-Chiari malformation, cancer, Crohn's disease, chronic pain, debilitating muscle spasms, glaucoma, hepatitis C, hydrocephalus, interstitial cystitis, lupus, multiple sclerosis, muscular dystrophy, neurofibromatosis, Parkinson's disease, PTSD, rheumatoid arthritis, seizures (including those characteristic of epilepsy), severe fibromyalgia, Sjogrens syndrome, spinal cord disease or injury, Tourette syndrome; traumatic brain injury, and wasting syndrome. The drug may also be used for end-of-life care.

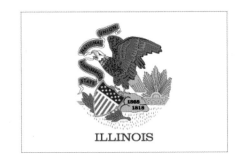

ILLINOIS

Louisiana

Louisiana is new to legalization and is still in the process of working out the details of their medical marijuana laws, but included so far are cancer, HIV/AIDS, seizure disorders, Crohn's disease, Parkinson's disease, muscular dystrophy, multiple sclerosis, PTSD, severe pain, and certain types of autism disorders.

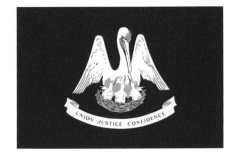

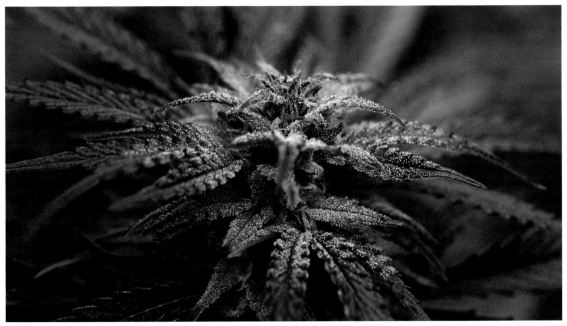

Maine

Cancer, glaucoma, HIV/AIDS, hepatitis C, ALS, Crohn's disease, Alzheimer's disease, PTSD, inflammatory bowel disease, cerebral palsy, intractable pain, and chronic or debilitating diseases or medical conditions that produce wasting syndrome, severe nausea, seizures (including epilepsy), or severe and persistent muscle spasms (including multiple sclerosis) are included in Maine's medical marijuana laws.

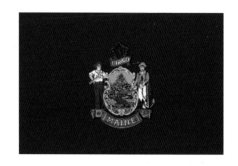

Maryland

Maryland's laws state that cannabis can be used to treat "any condition that is severe, for which other medical treatments have been ineffective, and if the symptoms reasonably can be expected to be relieved by the medical use of cannabis." The drug can also be used for glaucoma and PTSD, or if a patient has a chronic or debilitating disease or medical condition that causes severe loss of appetite, wasting syndrome, severe or chronic pain, severe nausea, seizures or severe or persistent muscle spasms.

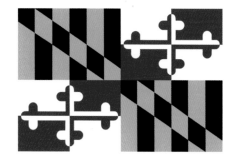

Massachusetts

Cancer, glaucoma, HIV/AIDS, hepatitis C, ALS, Crohn's disease, Parkinson's disease, and multiple sclerosis are all included. Other conditions may qualify if a patient's physician recommends cannabis in writing.

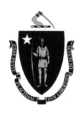

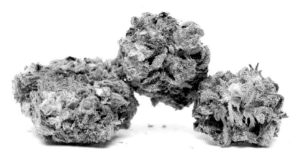

Michigan

In Michigan, cannabis is approved for treatment of cancer, glaucoma, HIV/AIDS, hepatitis C, ALS, Crohn's disease, Alzheimer's disease, wasting syndrome, severe and chronic pain, severe nausea, seizures, epilepsy, muscle spasms, multiple sclerosis, and PTSD.

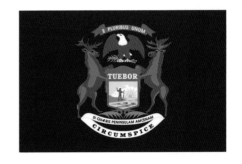

Minnesota

Cancer, glaucoma, HIV/AIDS, Tourette syndrome, ALS, seizures/epilepsy, severe and persistent muscle spasms, multiple sclerosis, Crohn's disease, terminal illness with a life expectancy of under one year, PTSD, intractable pain, and obstructive sleep apnea are all included, as well as certain autism disorders. Minnesota law does not allow marijuana to be smoked as a method of consumption.

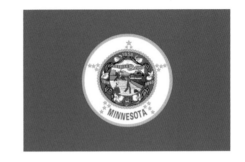

Montana

Montana's laws cover cancer, glaucoma, HIV/AIDS, or the treatment of these conditions; chronic or debilitating diseases or medical conditions or treatments that produce wasting syndrome, severe or chronic pain, severe nausea, seizures (including seizures caused by epilepsy), or severe or persistent muscle spasms (including spasms caused by multiple sclerosis or Crohn's disease); admittance to hospice care; painful peripheral neuropathy, central nervous system disorders resulting in chronic, painful spasticity or muscle spasms, and PTSD.

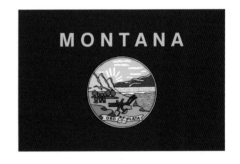

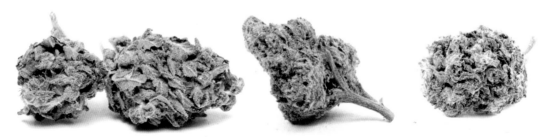

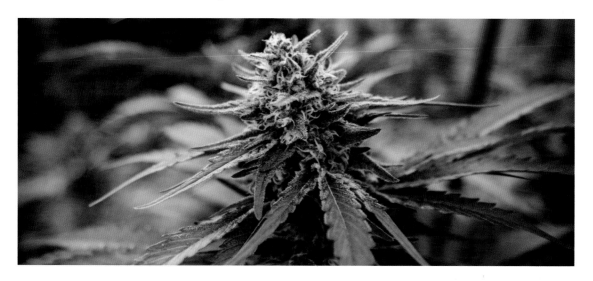

Nevada

HIV/AIDS, cancer, glaucoma, and any medical condition or treatment that produces wasting syndrome, persistent muscle spasms (including multiple sclerosis) or seizures (including epilepsy), severe nausea or pain, and PTSD are covered. Other conditions are subject to approval by the health division of the Nevada State Department of Human Resources.

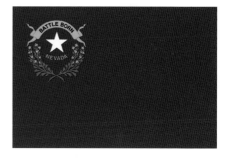

New Hampshire

New Hampshire allows the use of cannabis for cancer, glaucoma, HIV/AIDS, hepatitis C, ALS, muscular dystrophy, Crohn's disease, multiple sclerosis, PTSD, chronic pancreatitis, spinal cord injury or disease, traumatic brain injury, epilepsy, lupus, Parkinson's disease, Alzheimer's disease, or one or more injuries that significantly interfere with daily activities as documented by the patient's physician. Also covered are severely debilitating or terminal medical conditions or treatments that have produced at least one of the following: elevated intraocular pressure, chemotherapy-induced anorexia, wasting syndrome, agitation of Alzheimer's disease, severe pain that has not favorably responded to medication or surgical measures, constant or severe nausea, moderate to severe vomiting, seizures, or severe, persistent muscle spasms.

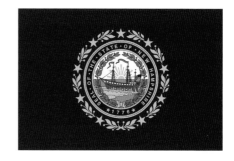

New Jersey

New Jersey's laws cover ALS, multiple sclerosis, terminal cancer, muscular dystrophy, inflammatory bowel disease (including Crohn's disease), terminal illness (if the physician has determined a prognosis of less than twelve months of life), chronic pain, anxiety, migraines, and Tourette syndrome. Cannabis may also be used for seizure disorders, muscle spasms, glaucoma, and PTSD if conventional therapies have been unsuccessful, and for HIV/AIDS and cancer if severe or chronic pain, severe nausea or vomiting, or wasting syndrome results from the condition or treatment.

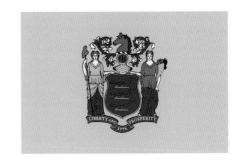

New Mexico

ALS, cancer, Crohn's disease, epilepsy, glaucoma, hepatitis C infection currently receiving antiviral treatment, HIV/AIDS, Huntington's Disease, hospice care, inflammatory muscle disease and autoimmune-mediated arthritis, intractable nausea/vomiting, multiple sclerosis, spinal cord injury, painful peripheral neuropathy, Parkinson's disease, PTSD, severe chronic pain, severe anorexia, spasmodic torticollis, and ulcerative colitis are all covered.

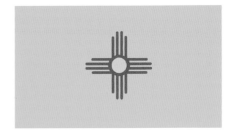

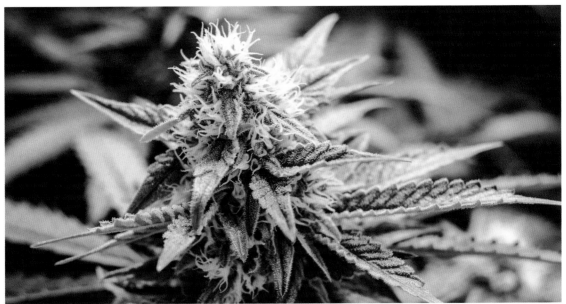

New York

In New York, medical marijuana may be used for cancer, HIV/AIDS, ALS, Parkinson's disease, multiple sclerosis, spinal cord injuries, epilepsy, inflammatory bowel disease, neuropathy, and Huntington's disease when the conditions are complicated by wasting syndrome, severe or chronic pain, severe nausea, seizures, or severe or persistent muscle spasms. Smoking is not an approved form of cannabis consumption in the state.

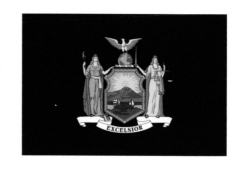

North Dakota

Cancer, HIV/AIDS, hepatitis C, ALS, PTSD, Alzheimer's disease, dementia, Crohn's disease, fibromyalgia, spinal stenosis or chronic back pain including neuropathy or damage to the nervous tissue of the spinal cord, glaucoma, and epilepsy are all included. Also included are any chronic or debilitating medical conditions or treatments that produce one or more of the following: wasting syndrome, severe debilitating pain that does not respond to medication or surgical treatment, intractable nausea, seizures, or severe and persistent muscle spasms (including those characteristic of multiple sclerosis). Any other medical condition must be approved by the North Dakota Department of Health.

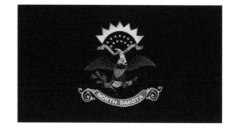

Ohio

AIDS/HIV, Alzheimer's disease, ALS, cancer, chronic traumatic encephalopathy, Crohn's disease, epilepsy, fibromyalgia, glaucoma, hepatitis C, inflammatory bowel disease, multiple sclerosis, chronic severe pain, Parkinson's disease, PTSD, sickle cell anemia, spinal cord disease or injury, Tourette syndrome, traumatic brain injury, and ulcerative colitis are included in Ohio's laws. Smoking marijuana is not approved.

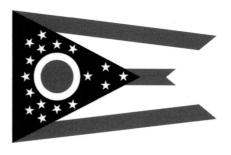

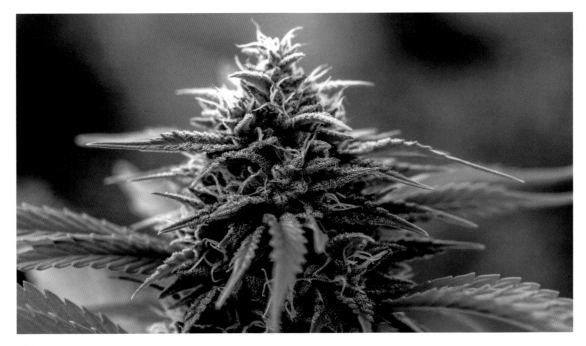

Oregon

Oregon allows medical marijuana use for cancer, glaucoma, degenerative or pervasive neurological conditions, and HIV/AIDS, as well as any medical conditions or treatments that produce wasting syndrome, severe pain, severe nausea, seizures (including seizures caused by epilepsy), or persistent muscle spasms (including spasms caused by multiple sclerosis). Other conditions are subject to approval by the Health Division of the Oregon Department of Human Resources.

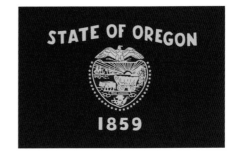

Pennsylvania

Pennsylvania's cannabis laws cover cancer, HIV/AIDS, ALS, Parkinson's, multiple sclerosis, spinal cord disease or injury, epilepsy, inflammatory bowel disease, neuropathies, Huntington's disease, Crohn's disease, PTSD, intractable seizures, glaucoma, sickle cell anemia, severe chronic pain which does not respond to conventional treatment, and certain autism disorders. Smoking is not an approved form of consumption.

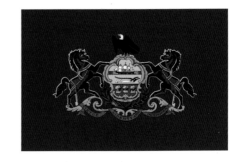

Rhode Island

Included in Rhode Island's medical marijuana laws are cancer, glaucoma, HIV/AIDS, and hepatitis C. Also included are any chronic or debilitating diseases or medical conditions or treatments that produce wasting syndrome; severe, debilitating, chronic pain; severe nausea; seizures (including those characteristic of epilepsy); or severe and persistent muscle spasms (including those characteristic of multiple sclerosis or Crohn's disease); or agitation of Alzheimer's Disease. Other medical conditions may be approved by the Rhode Island Department of Health.

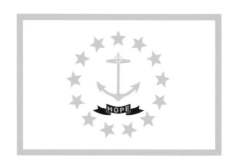

Vermont

Cancer, HIV/AIDS, multiple sclerosis, and glaucoma are covered under Vermont's laws, including the treatment of the aforementioned conditions if the treatment results in severe, persistent, and intractable symptoms. Also covered are any diseases, medical conditions, or treatments that are chronic and debilitating and produce severe and persistent symptoms such as wasting syndrome, chronic pain, nausea, or seizures.

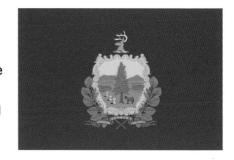

Washington

In the state of Washington, medical marijuana laws cover cancer, HIV/AIDS, multiple sclerosis, epilepsy or other seizure disorder, intractable pain (limited to pain unrelieved by standard medical treatments and medications), glaucoma, Crohn's disease with debilitating symptoms unrelieved by standard treatments or medications, PTSD, traumatic brain injury, and hepatitis C with debilitating nausea or intractable pain unrelieved by standard treatments or medications. Also covered are diseases which result in nausea, vomiting, wasting syndrome, appetite loss, cramping, seizures, muscle spasms, or spasticity, when these symptoms are unrelieved by standard treatments or medications.

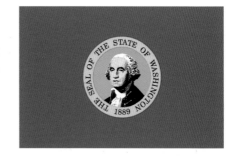

Washington, D.C.

Medical cannabis laws in the nation's capital cover HIV/AIDS, cancer, glaucoma, conditions characterized by severe and persistent muscle spasms (such as multiple sclerosis), patients undergoing chemotherapy or radiotherapy, severe liver cirrhosis, ALS, wasting syndrome, Alzheimer's disease, and seizure disorders.

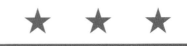

West Virginia

Conditions covered under West Virginia's medical cannabis laws are subject to approval by the West Virginia Medical Cannabis Commission. These include chronic or debilitating diseases or medical conditions that result in hospice care or palliative care, and chronic or debilitating diseases or medical conditions or the treatment of chronic or debilitating diseases or medical conditions that result in: wasting syndrome or anorexia; severe or chronic pain that does not find effective relief through standard pain medication; severe nausea; seizures; severe or persistent muscle spasms; refractory generalized anxiety disorder; or PTSD. The state does not allow smoking marijuana as a method of consumption.

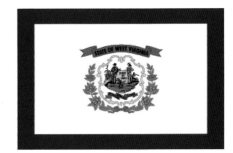

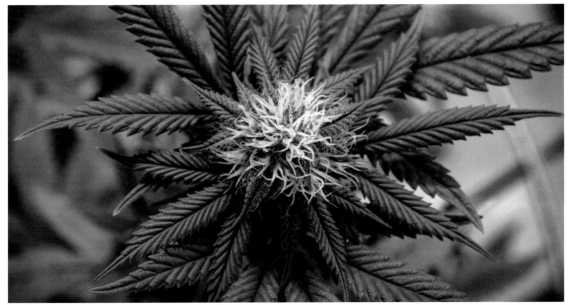

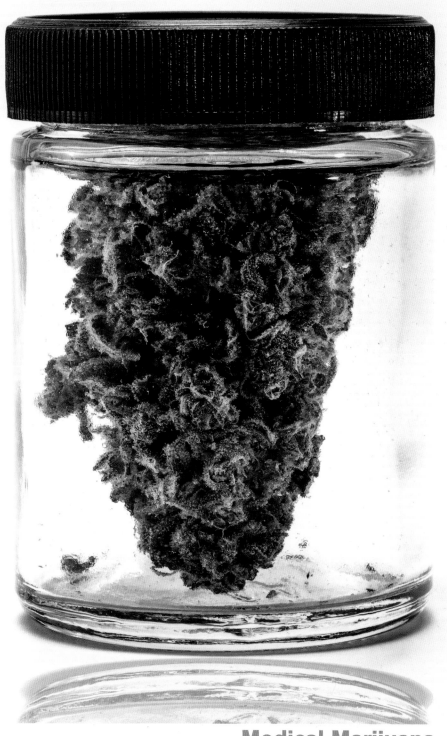

Why Marijuana?

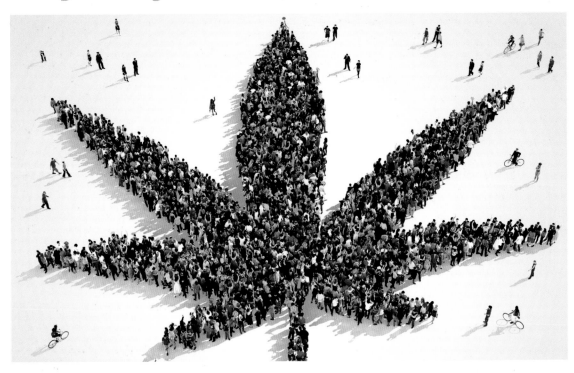

In this day and age, we are bombarded with advertisements for new drugs on what seems like a daily basis. Television commercials, magazine ads, and internet popups constantly remind us to talk to our doctors about our ailments and the possible miraculous cures offered by the pharmaceutical industry. With so many drug choices on the market, you'd think that every possible malady would have a corresponding option to fight unpleasant symptoms.

But even with literally thousands of drugs on the market, finding a perfect match for your symptoms isn't always easy. Some people try drug after drug without success, leaving them feeling as if they've reached the end of their rope. As we can see from the previous list of ailments covered by medical marijuana laws in many states, this is where marijuana can often step in to help.

The Right Drug?

Consider the current opioid epidemic in the United States: in the 1990s, doctors began prescribing more and more opioid painkillers to patients—drugs such as hydrocodone, oxycodone, and fentanyl. But it soon became apparent that these drugs were, in fact, highly addictive, and abuse of opioids has risen ever since. Presently, more than one hundred people die in the U.S. due to opioid overdose every day, and nearly a quarter of patients prescribed the drugs end up misusing them.

If cannabis was a legal alternative, patients with chronic, unrelenting pain would have another choice to ease symptoms besides highly addictive opioids. In fact, in states that have legalized medical marijuana, opioid use is already dropping. A study published in *JAMA: The Journal of the American Medical Association* in May 2018 found that among those who use Medicare, opioid use dropped fourteen percent in states with access to medical marijuana. This is an estimated reduction of 3.7 million daily doses of opioids. While the study isn't necessarily definitive proof, as it shows only a correlation between lower opioid use and legal medical marijuana states, the two do seem to be connected: Prescriptions for medications to treat anxiety, nausea,

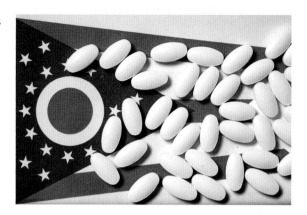

In 2017, Ohio had the second highest rate of opioid overdose deaths in the U.S. after West Virginia, according to the Center of Disease Control and Prevention. Between the years 2015 and 2016 there was a thirty percent increase in deaths caused by overdoses in Ohio. As research continues to study the medicinal effects of marijuana, hopefully these stats begin to decrease.

and seizures (all of which marijuana has been shown to help) also dropped, whereas prescriptions for blood thinners (which cannot be replaced with marijuana) remained the same in these states. And since marijuana is far less addictive than opioids and does not cause overdoses, it could help save some of the thousands of lives lost to opioid overdoses every year. This is not to say that marijuana is without risks—all drugs have the potential to be abused—but the research clearly shows that medicinal cannabis could be a viable alternative to the frightening opioid epidemic in this country.

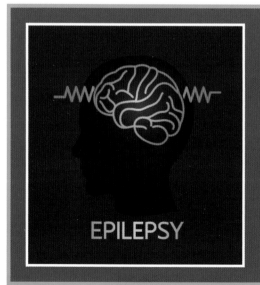

EPILEPSY

Epilepsy and Marijuana

A study from the Stanford University Medical Center on treatment-resistant pediatric epilepsy patients found that twelve different anti-epilepsy medications were not successful in controlling seizures. Out of nineteen epilepsy patients, sixteen exhibited reduced numbers of seizures after beginning treatment with cannabis. So after an average of a dozen failed conventional drug attempts, medical cannabis ended up showing the most promise. As CNN's Chief Medical Correspondent Dr. Sanjay Gupta said in a 2013 column on CNN.com, "Sometimes, marijuana is the only thing that works."

Getting Carded

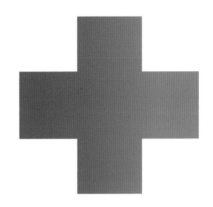

Now that thirty states (and counting) have legalized marijuana for medicinal use, it's easier than ever for Americans to obtain cannabis. But before you can walk into a dispensary and buy a cannabis product, you'll need to have a medical marijuana card. This card protects individuals from civil and criminal penalties in states without laws for recreational use. But gaining a card isn't as easy as simply asking your doctor for one; there are a few steps you'll need to take to procure access to medical marijuana.

Knowing What's Covered

First, of course, you should be familiar with the marijuana laws in your own state. Those who live in cannabis-averse Idaho, for instance, are unable to obtain medical marijuana for any reason. If you're certain your state has medical marijuana laws, you'll need to find out which conditions and diseases are approved for treatment with medicinal cannabis.

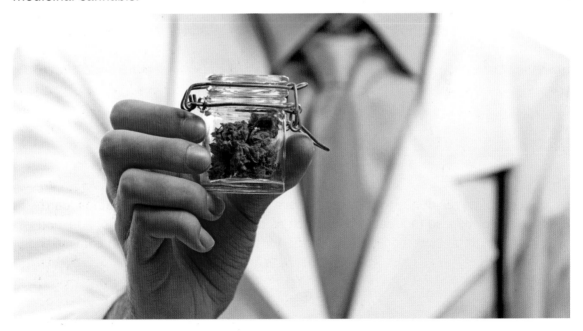

Some states may also require doctors to be specially registered with the department of health in order to recommend marijuana—if your doctor is not registered, ask to be referred to someone who is.

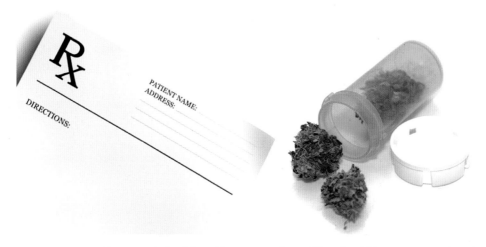

Your state's health and human services office should have a comprehensive
list of conditions covered for treatment with marijuana.

Talking To Your Doctor

Once you know that your condition is approved for medical marijuana, you'll need to get a
physician recommendation. This step can be tricky, since not all doctors are convinced that
marijuana can be used as a therapeutic remedy. Arm yourself with as much information
as you can, to bolster the case for cannabis. If your doctor is particularly hesitant, you
may need to shop around for a more open-minded physician; a doctor's recommendation
is crucial to obtaining a medical card. Some states have made this step much easier,
however, by providing a list of doctors who are certified to recommend marijuana to
patients. Check online to familiarize yourself with your state's medical marijuana process
and look for suggestions to find a cannabis-friendly doctor. And no matter what channel
you go through to find a doctor, be sure to always have your medical records handy to
make the process move along more quickly.

The next step is to fill out a patient application. This is also when you will need to
provide proof of residency in the state where you are obtaining the medical card.
Many applications also require a photo (such as a passport photo), proof of age, and
an agreement to be fingerprinted. Caregivers for those who are unable to administer
their own cannabis may also be asked to fill out an application and provide fingerprints.
Finally, be prepared to pay a fee—the cost is usually between fifty and one-hundred
dollars for a one-year medical marijuana card, although the fee may be lower for
veterans or for those who are eligible for disability. Caregivers may also be asked to
pay a modest fee, usually around twenty-five dollars. And don't forget to renew your
card when it nears the expiration date—you'll likely need to reapply to obtain a new one.

Recreational Marijuana States

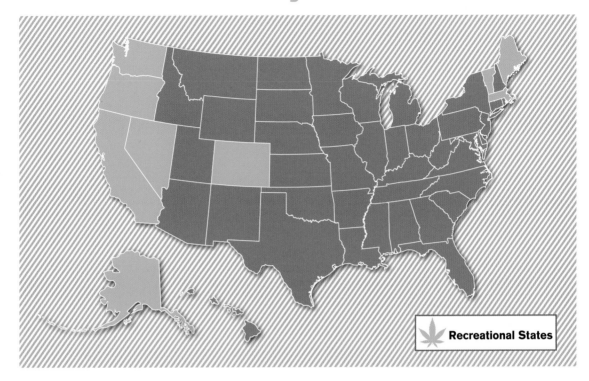

Recreational States

We've seen the states that have legalized marijuana for medicinal purposes, so now let's look at the states that have taken things one step further and legalized the drug for recreational use, as well. These states include Alaska, California, Colorado, Maine, Massachusetts, Nevada, Oregon, Vermont, Washington, and Washington, D.C.

Most of these states allow users to possess up to one ounce of marijuana, although Washington, D.C., allows two ounces, and Maine allows two and a half. Oregon allows one ounce in public, but up to eight ounces in a user's home. Most of these states also allow personal cultivation of the plant, with limits. Maine allows up to fifteen plants (but only three of those plants can be mature), while Oregon allows four plants. Most of the other states allow up to six plants, with the exception of Washington state, where growing any number of plants is illegal; however, if it's needed for medicinal purposes, Washington residents may be eligible for a grower's license.

The Upside
Proponents of cannabis collectively cheer every time another state legalizes the drug for recreational use. And not just because it gives more people the freedom to use marijuana if they choose. Legalizing cannabis has had some great upsides in the states that have done so. For instance, in Colorado's first year of selling legalized cannabis, the state brought in

$700 million in sales. In only the first month of Nevada's legal sales, the state sold $27 million and brought in $3.6 million in tax revenue. Oregon has paid out $85 million in tax revenue from marijuana sales to help fund schools, public health initiatives, and emergency services. And since the drug was legalized in Washington in 2014, sales have topped $1 billion, with sales taxes exceeding $250 million for the state.

And these states don't just bring in money from sales of marijuana—they also bring in tourist dollars. Cannabis tourism has been a growing industry in recent years, thanks to newly legalized locales and the out-of-state visitors who want to experience them. In 2016, a Colorado tourism survey found that fifteen percent of visitors to the state participated in some kind of marijuana-related activity while they were there. And when they're not visiting a dispensary or taking a cannabis tour, these tourists spend money in the state's hotels, restaurants, and shops. Marijuana-friendly travel companies will even help plan a getaway: Companies like CannabisTours.com—which plans trips in Denver, Las Vegas, Washington, D.C., Portland, Boston, and throughout California—can suggest marijuana-friendly hotels, book classes and activities, and can take visitors on a party-bus tour around the city to see marijuana cultivation facilities (with, of course, a chance to sample the merchandise). And in Alaska, marijuana store owners have begun opening shop within walking distance of the cruise ship docks that bring in more than a million passengers each year. It's easy to see that the recreational legalization of marijuana has had some positive effects on the states that have chosen to legalize.

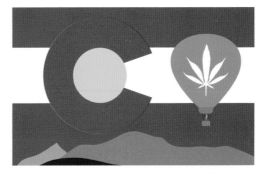

Colorado's Amendment 64, which passed on November 6, 2012, and was enacted in January of 2014, has led to many positive results for the state's economic, political, and cultural institutions. Colorado collected $247 million in taxes, fees, and licensing costs in 2017 alone.

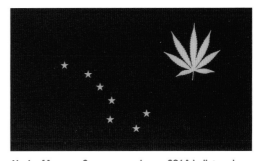

Alaska Measure 2 was passed on a 2014 ballot and was enacted on February 24, 2015, legalizing the recreational use of marijuana in the state. The first month of tax revenue from recreational marijuana garnered the state of Alaska $80,000.

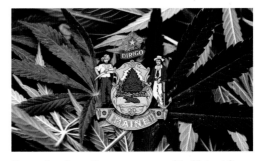

Recreational marijuana was passed in Maine after voters enacted to pass Maine Question 1, 2016. The law imposes a ten percent tax on the commercial sales of recreational marijuana and also allows for onsite consumption at locations that are licensed for it.

How to Find a Dispensary

Years ago, the options for purchasing a bit of cannabis were pretty limited. You could either surreptitiously buy some from a random dealer—maybe a kid behind the high school gym or an adventurous soccer mom in the grocery store parking lot—or you could travel to a location where the substance was legal. But flying all the way to Amsterdam just for some marijuana seems like quite a bit of trouble. Fortunately, options these days are much more out in the open, and certainly closer to home. But if you're unfamiliar with dispensaries nearby, how do you find a good location? These days, we can look no further than the internet.

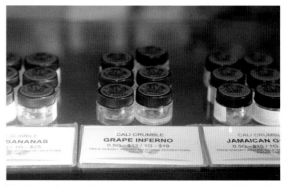

Marijuana dispensaries are surprisingly sophisticated. You will find a number of products and strains you can choose from and a helpful employee working the counter, which is much different from the shady situations that most marijuana users encountered before the laws around the plant were relaxed.

A great place to start your search is at Leafly.com. This Seattle-based, cannabis-friendly website not only lists every dispensary nearby, but it also plots them on a map and shows user reviews, so you can browse pros and cons. Clicking on a specific dispensary will also bring up a list of products that a particular dispensary carries, including buds and flowers, waxes and oils, and edibles. The site also allows you to browse the strains that are available at each dispensary according to price, CBD or THC content, or brand name, so you can find one that meets your specific needs.

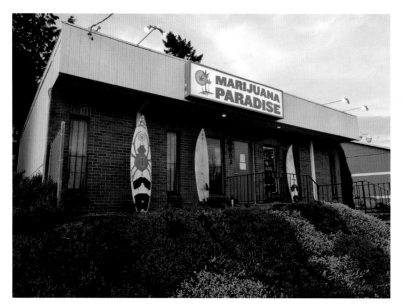

Dispensaries are not ashamed of their businesses and can often be found in high-traffic shopping areas in states where marijuana has been made legal.

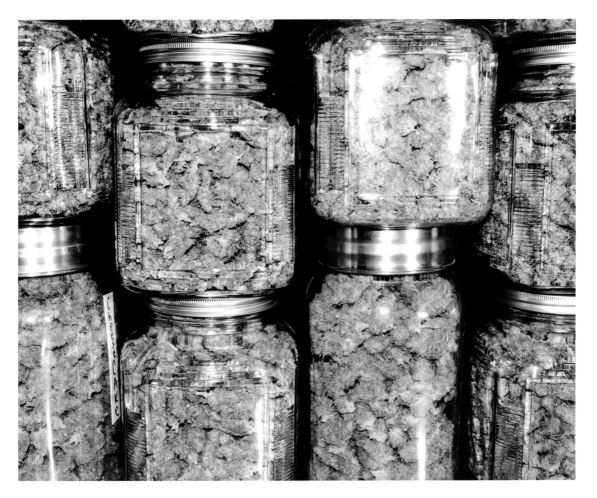

With the legalization of marijuana, the quality, consistency, and variety will continue to get better as prices continue to become more manageable.

Alternately, you can begin browsing through strains using filters to narrow your search according to symptoms, conditions, desired effects, or even flavors. Leafly.com will then bring up a list of strains, and the dispensary locations near you that sell them.

The website publishes a regular "Leafly List" which details the highest-ranking dispensaries in different locations around the country. So you can always stay up to date on the best dispensary locations in the country. With 20,000 dispensary reviews and 50,000 strain reviews, Leafly.com is often called "the Yelp of weed." Their connoisseur-like approach to marijuana—not unlike foodies who review restaurants or chocoholics who revel in the perfect truffle—caters to recreational and medical users alike. If you're confused about where to start in your search, this website is the perfect beginner resource.

Marijuana vs. Big Business

As research into cannabis and demand for the drug continues, more and more states are moving to legalize the plant, either for medicinal or recreational use. The industry is literally growing like a weed (pardon the pun)!

It's obvious that cannabis legalization comes with some pros—an influx of tax dollars, more jobs, and a boost to the economy. But some worry about cons, as well. Recently, our neighbor to the north passed the Cannabis Act, which will legalize marijuana for recreational use for adults throughout Canada. But many Canadians worry about the lack of regulations in place for the industry. For instance, there are no clear guidelines in place for driving under the influence of marijuana, unlike alcohol.

Some Possible Downfalls

Another concern is the existence of the marijuana black market. In places where the drug is not legal, black market dealers are able to make quite a profit for themselves, without having to worry about paying for a storefront or dealing with taxes. Will these dealers be willing to legitimatize their businesses and go through legal channels? And if not, will their prices be low enough that consumers will forgo the legal businesses and continue to buy cannabis on the black market?

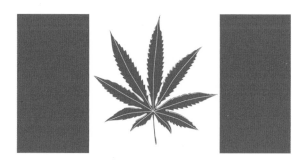

Already in Canada, a mere eight growers are poised to take control of seventy percent of the country's cannabis production by 2021.

One other issue that concerns many about cannabis legalization is the influence of big business on the industry. As marijuana becomes more popular and accepted, smaller shops and growers will be replaced with larger businesses, when investors rush to get in on the booming commodity. Already in Canada, a mere eight growers are poised to take control of seventy percent of the country's cannabis production by 2021.

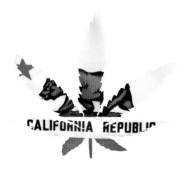

In cannabis-legal California, twenty percent of the 697 total marijuana cultivation licenses belonged to just twelve businesses.

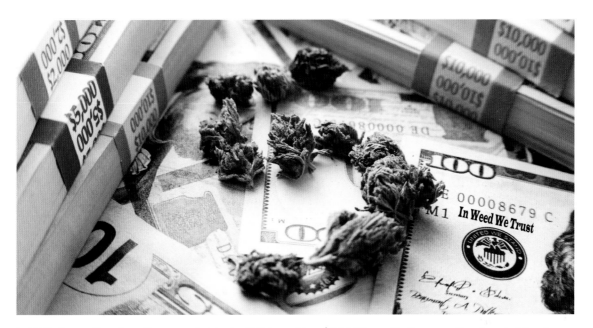

In 2017, the medicinal marijuana market in the U.S. brought in $5.3 billion, with the recreational market topping out at $2.6 billion. And those numbers are expected to grow: By 2025, the cannabis industry is expected to bring in about $24 billion total, and could create as many as 300,000 new jobs.

Some Possible Upsides

But this big-business cannabis takeover isn't necessarily a bad thing. Larger growers are able to keep their costs lower, which in turn means cheaper cannabis for consumers. Take the state of Washington, for instance: When marijuana was first legalized in the state in 2014, wholesalers could buy a gram of cannabis for eight dollars. Then big business swooped in and bulked up capacity with state-of-the-art technology, resulting in cheaper cannabis for all. As of 2017, a gram of the drug cost less than three dollars.

These big businesses, of course, run the risk of driving smaller merchants out of the market. But lower costs may also drive out black market dealers, who can't afford to sell their products cheaply. There are always pros and cons to any endeavor; for now, we'll have to keep a close eye on our Canadian neighbors and take notes.

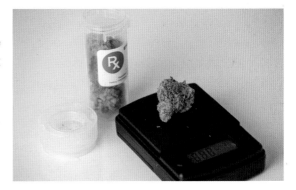

Black market marijuana prices are inflated to cover the risk dealers take in order to provide their illegal service. But when legalization of medical and recreational marijuana happens on a larger scale, prices will continue to drop as production cost drops.

Don't Get Testy

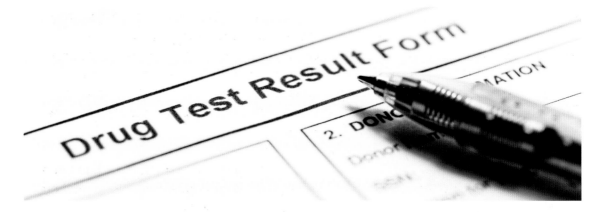

Say you're eager to land a new job at a big company: You do your research into the corporation, get called in for an interview, and make a fantastic first impression. They decide you're the perfect candidate for the job; you can't wait to pick up your employee ID card from human resources on your first day. All that remains is a simple drug test. And then you find out that the test detected marijuana, even though the last time you ingested the drug was more than a week ago. But because your new company has a "zero tolerance" policy, they move on to the next candidate.

How Does It Work?

So why was the test positive in the first place? After all, the effects of cannabis only last a few hours. In fact, THC is only detectable in blood for a few hours, so blood tests are often used to test for sobriety after automobile accidents or other times when impairment is suspected. But once the substance leaves the bloodstream, it is broken down into molecules known as metabolites, which are stored in body fat and gradually eliminated over time. This is why traces of THC can be found in urine tests days—or even weeks—after using marijuana. Urine tests (which are what most employers use to test for drugs) can only show that cannabis has been used—they don't indicate intoxication or impairment of any kind. Regardless, this means that even if you use marijuana only on your own time—even in states where it is legal—an employer with a workplace drug policy may terminate employees who test positive.

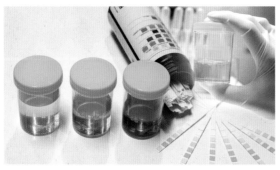

The confusing laws have prompted many to try creative techniques to "fool" drug tests. Some of these include drinking lots of water to "flush" THC from the system; adding bleach, salt, or detergent to urine samples; or using special "cleansing" herbal teas. But none of these is a reliable way to pass a drug test.

The Legal Confusion

This may seem like an unfair situation considering cannabis is now legal in so many states, whether for recreational or medicinal use. But many employers have decided to conduct business as usual—meaning, their policies are exactly the same as they were prior to marijuana legalization. Take California, for instance: The state legalized recreational marijuana use under Prop 64 at the beginning of 2018, but according to the Los Angeles Times, Prop 64 "does not change the legal status between employers and employees when it comes to drug testing and employment."

Compounding the problem is that many people assume that if marijuana has been legalized in their state, their occasional weekend use should have no bearing on their employment. But unfortunately, cannabis legalization has created a bit of a gray area for usage: Yes, you may be legally allowed to use marijuana in your state, but your employer is also allowed to create a drug policy that prohibits that use.

A Guaranteed Way to Pass

The bottom line is, if your employer has a "zero tolerance" policy when it comes to drugs, the only guaranteed way to pass a drug test is to avoid cannabis in the weeks leading up to the test. This includes everything from smoking to edibles. But things may soon be changing: Recently, the Fairness in Federal Drug Testing Under State Laws Act (H.R. 6589) was introduced to Congress, which would protect employees who test positive for marijuana in states where the drug is legal, but would still prohibit intoxication at work. Although the bill would only apply to federal employees, it is a step toward ending employers' interference in employees' private lives. And who knows—maybe it will be an end to the fake urine business, as well!

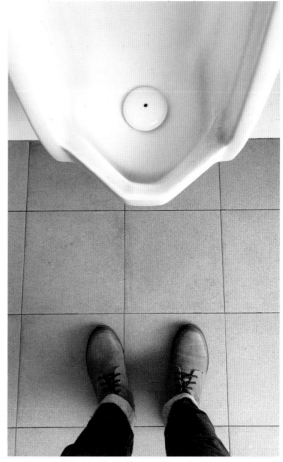

It's possible for synthetic urine to fool a test—yes, a fake urine market actually exists—but it's a risky endeavor to attempt a urine switcheroo during a drug test. Testing is becoming more sensitive as well—synthetic urine will have to keep up with the newest technology if it wants to keep passing for the real thing.

Keeping Kids Safe

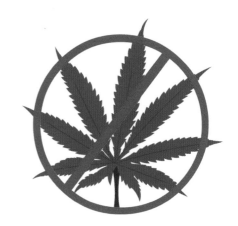

There are so many benefits that cannabis can provide to those who are sick or suffering, and the drug has many upsides: It's relatively safe, it has few side effects, and an overdose is almost impossible. But it's important to remember that cannabis is still a drug — and just like any drug, there are concerns and dangers that come along with its usage. And nowhere are those concerns more valid than when it comes to children.

The Risks

One of the myths about marijuana is that it is never addictive. This isn't true—in fact, about one in ten adults becomes addicted to the substance, and can require assistance to break the habit. But the risk for addiction is even greater for children: Teenagers who use marijuana have a forty percent chance of developing an addiction. And new studies are suggesting that cannabis use in adolescence can disrupt brain development, adding another hazard to teenage addiction.

Another concern is that a parent's marijuana use—just like alcohol use—can be a factor when it comes to child custody or neglect cases, even in states where the drug is legal. Some children have been removed from homes because cannabis products have been stored in locations within reach, sometimes causing accidental ingestion.

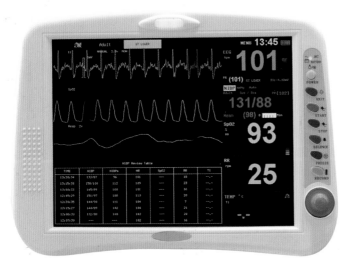

In Colorado in 2014, when cannabis was recreationally legalized in the state, emergency rooms saw twice as many children for accidental cannabis ingestion as they saw before it was legalized. The majority of these resulted in only minor health effects, but fourteen percent of these children experienced racing heart rate, respiratory distress, low blood pressure, or seizures.

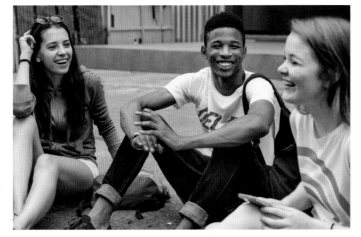

Despite the well-founded worry and concern over cannabis use by young people, there is good news: Even with recent recreational legalization in several states, there has not been an increase in marijuana usage among teenagers. Regardless, it's always smart to do all we can to keep children and teenagers safe and healthy, and preventing accidental ingestion or intentional abuse of cannabis products is a must for responsible consumers.

How to Keep Kids Safe

When it comes to young children, tips for preventing cannabis ingestion are much the same as any other drug or alcohol. For instance, always keep cannabis out of reach and out of sight of curious children. This is especially important for cannabis edibles, as brownies, candy, gummy bears, and other snacks can be irresistible to kids. Always make sure to return cannabis products to their safe location, every single time they're used. Investing in a lock box can be a great way to securely store marijuana products and other medications, and parents should talk to their kids about how these drugs need to be consumed safely and should only be handled by adults.

In this day and age of increasing legal recreational use, it's always good to speak to other adults who may visit your home, and request that they keep any cannabis products out of reach of children as well. The same goes for homes that children visit—it may seem strange to ask other parents about their marijuana usage, but with the popularity of cannabis ever increasing, it's not such a stretch to assume that other responsible adults may be using the drug now and then.

Teenagers who use marijuana often first try the drug around age fourteen; so it's important to talk to kids about cannabis long before they're given a chance to try it. And of course, staying involved in teenagers' lives, setting clear guidelines, and always keeping the lines of communication open are important steps. Researchers also have other suggestions for keeping marijuana out of the hands of young people. One is to keep cannabis prices relatively high, since most teenagers are especially concerned with money. In fact, studies have shown that teens who smoke cigarettes are more likely to curb their use when prices are raised; high-priced marijuana products may not look as attractive to a teenager who's saving up for a smartphone or a car. Researchers also suggest maintaining tight control on retail shops that sell cannabis products, enacting stiff penalties for shops that sell to minors.

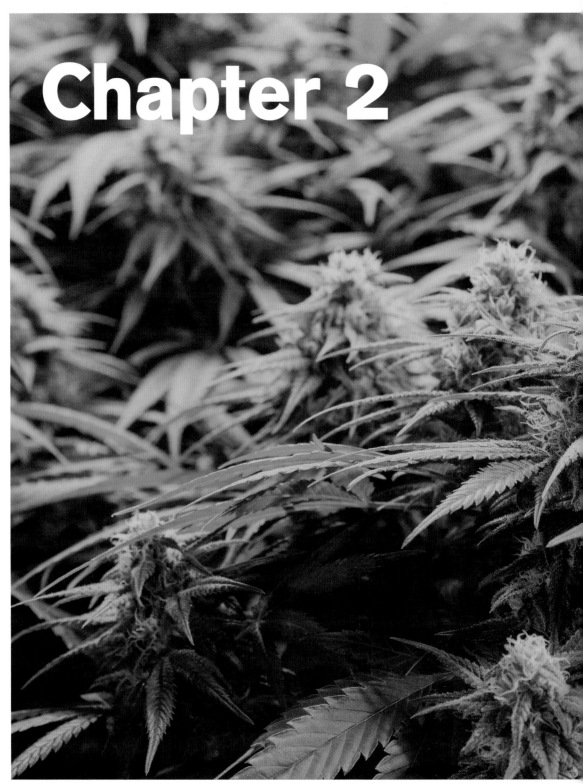

Chapter 2

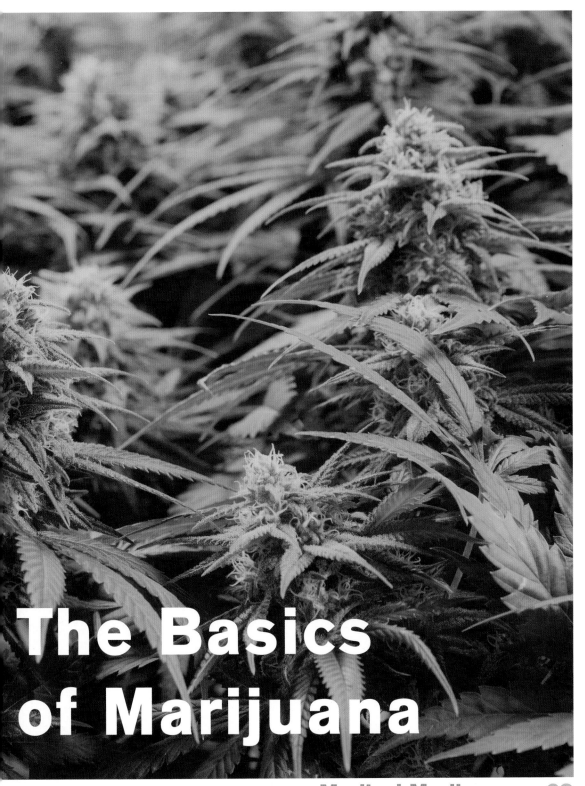

The Basics
of Marijuana

What Gives Marijuana Its High?

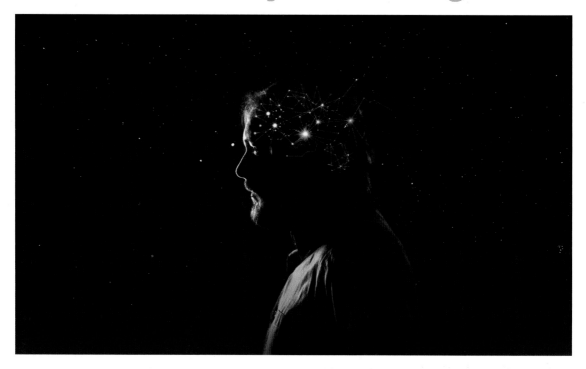

The endocannabinoid system, the endogenous biological system of cannabinoid receptors, is responsible for many important functions in the human body. In general it mostly regulates homeostasis within our body, guiding our mood, overall health, and the physiological effects and "high" of voluntary exercise. It is also the system that allows our body to process the pharmacological effects of cannabis.

Even if you've never tried marijuana (or, like Bill Clinton, you "didn't inhale") you've no doubt heard about how users of the drug experience a "high" when they consume it. People report everything from euphoria to anxiety to hallucinations when using cannabis, with effects lasting an average of two hours. The source of these effects is a chemical called tetrahydrocannabinol, or THC.

When ingested, THC is able to bind to molecules in the brain's endocannabinoid system, which is a neural communication network that helps to regulate many of the body's functions, including appetite, mood, memory, and pain, as well as physical movement. When the THC binds with the molecules in this system, it disrupts these functions in various ways. For example, THC may affect a person's ability to form short-term memories or perform complicated tasks, and may alter balance and slow reaction time. It can also activate the brain's reward system, flooding the brain with dopamine and producing feelings of euphoria.

The Receptors

The molecules that bind with the compounds in marijuana are receptors called CB1 and CB2. CB1 is mostly found in the brain—in fact, there are ten times as many CB1 receptors in the brain as there are opioid receptors responsible for the effects of morphine. THC causes the CB1 receptors to "over-activate," causing all kinds of psychological effects. Since everyone's body is different, everyone's "high" when using marijuana is different, as well. While some people experience euphoria and relaxation, others can feel anxious or paranoid.

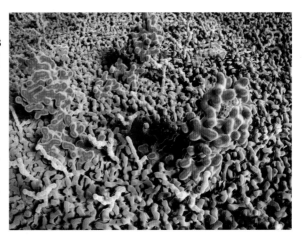

A 3D rendering of THC molecules binding to the CB1 receptor.

And THC doesn't only affect the brain—it also binds to receptors in other areas of the body, like the CB2 receptors that are found on the cells of the immune system. When THC binds with these receptors, it can have an anti-inflammatory effect, which is one of the reasons the drug is gaining popularity as a medicinal remedy. THC can also stimulate the release of the hormone ghrelin—also known as "the hunger hormone"—which gives marijuana its notorious reputation for causing "the munchies."

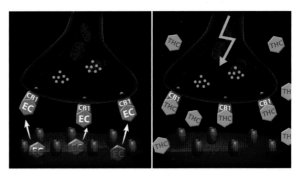

An illustration depicting the bonding that takes place at the CB1 receptor with both endogenous cannabinoids and THC.

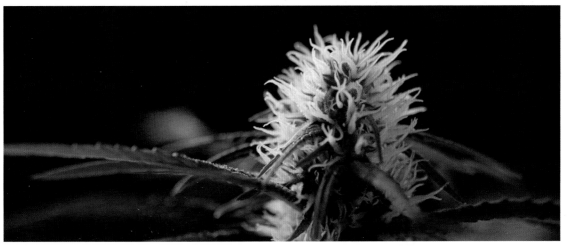

Benefits of THC

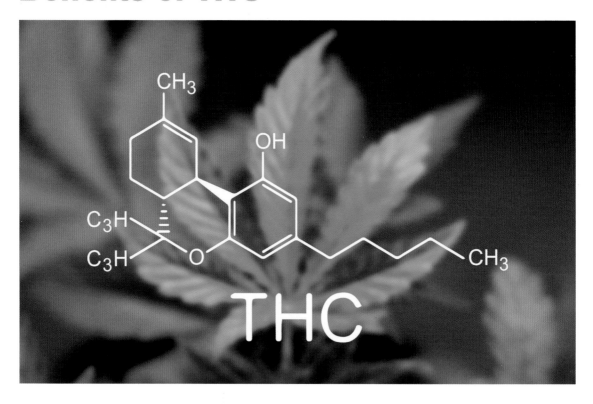

Euphoria and the munchies may seem like fun, but THC is far more than just a way to get "high." Many of its effects have been found to be beneficial—some of them in surprising ways.

Anti-Inflammation

THC's anti-inflammatory properties have made it an increasingly popular therapeutic treatment for a host of ailments, like autoimmune disorders and multiple sclerosis. Researchers have also started to investigate the chemical's effects on cancer cells, with some promising results: THC has been shown to shrink cancer tumors in laboratory animals and prevent cancer from metastasizing.

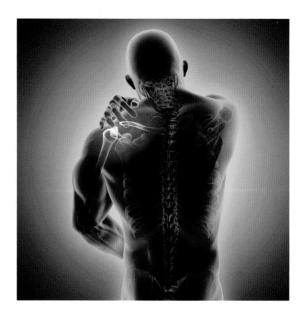

Dopamine

The chemical's ability to increase dopamine is just like that of opioids—but THC is much safer and far less addictive. Couple that with its anti-inflammatory properties, and it's easy to see why one of THC's most popular medicinal uses is as a pain reliever.

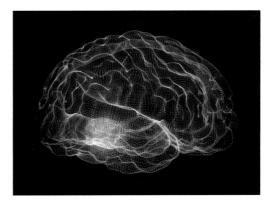

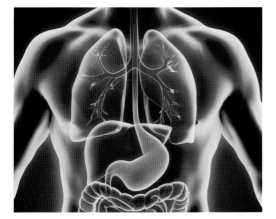

Increasing Appetite

And that reputation for causing "the munchies"? While it may not be great for anyone who's watching their weight, that urge to eat is very much a positive for those who suffer from digestive disorders or severe nausea due to chemotherapy or disease.

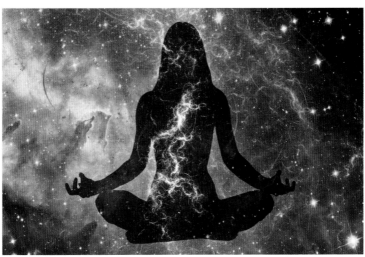

Easing Your Mind

Easing pain is obviously a positive for the drug, but it may seem like THC's propensity for influencing a user's short-term memory would be a less-than-desirable side effect. However, this response can actually be beneficial for some people. Researchers have found that cannabis can help those who are dealing with troubling memories, such as people suffering with PTSD, depression, or anxiety.

Benefits of CBD

As we've seen, THC binds with molecules in the brain's endocannabinoid system in order to produce its effects. The compounds that bind with the receptors in the endocannabinoid system are called, fittingly, cannabinoids. THC is just one of at least eighty-five cannabinoids found in the cannabis plant—and there may even be more than a hundred. Marijuana's cannabinoids are found in the trichromes—the shiny, sticky "hairs" on the flowers—of the plant.

While THC is the most talked-about cannabinoid in marijuana, because of its ability to cause a "high" and its medicinal properties, it is not the only one with benefits. Many of these compounds have yet to be studied in detail, and have tongue-twister names like cannabigerol, cannabinol, and cannabichromene. But another compound—cannabidiol, or CBD—is making headlines with its medicinal abilities, and some scientists think it could revolutionize medicine as we know it.

Sourcing and Accessing CBD

Unlike THC, CBD is not psychoactive—meaning it can't give you the "high" associated with THC. This is an important attribute, as it is the THC in marijuana—not the other compounds—that is considered illegal in some states. So when CBD is isolated on its own, it can work its way around the legal issues that entangle THC. Products containing CBD can easily be purchased in many stores or online. In fact, even the DEA has stated that curbing the use of CBD is not a priority. Still, the legality of marijuana in each state dictates where the CBD sold in that state comes from. If there are no medical cannabis laws in a state, CBD usually comes from low-to-no-THC hemp plants. But in states with medical cannabis laws, CBD can come from marijuana plants and, in some cases, can contain up to five percent THC.

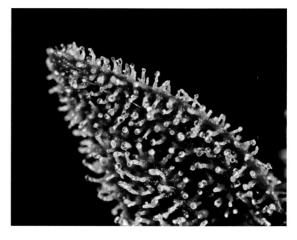

The female cannabis plant only begins to develop buds with sticky trichomes if it has not been pollinated by a male cannabis plant. The female plant will still produce trichomes if it is pollinated, but it will dedicate more energy to seed production rather than bud production.

The CBD Effect

One of the most promising effects CBD seems to have is as an anticonvulsant. Studies have shown that the compound works to prevent seizures and could be a great therapy for epilepsy. It has also been shown to have a "neuroprotective effect" which can prevent and treat neurological diseases like Alzheimer's, multiple sclerosis, and Parkinson's. Like THC, CBD has been shown to be a pain reliever, and it can also work together with morphine to counteract the opioid's side effects. CBD can slow the progression of cancer cells, reduce inflammation, and may help to treat mood disorders.

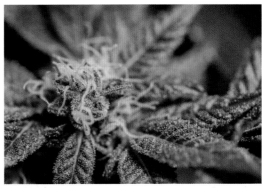

This strain of marijuana, ACDC, is a sativa-dominant strain that produces large amounts of CBD with a THC:CBD ratio of a 1:20. This plant does not create intoxicating effects and has CBD levels near nineteen percent. The plant helps patients in treating pain, epilepsy, and multiple sclerosis.

In addition to all of these, CBD provides one more benefit for those who choose to use marijuana recreationally: The compound actually acts as a counterweight to the psychoactive properties of THC, helping to reduce negative THC side-effects. For this reason, many cannabis users look for marijuana strains with a one to one THC/CBD ratio.

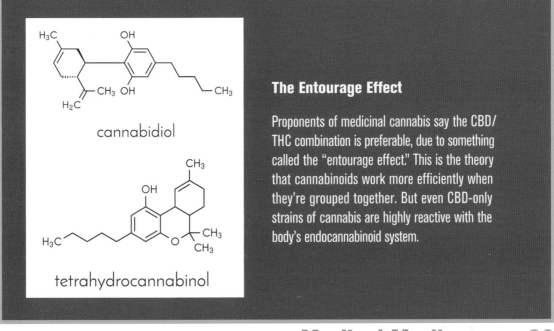

cannabidiol

tetrahydrocannabinol

The Entourage Effect

Proponents of medicinal cannabis say the CBD/THC combination is preferable, due to something called the "entourage effect." This is the theory that cannabinoids work more efficiently when they're grouped together. But even CBD-only strains of cannabis are highly reactive with the body's endocannabinoid system.

A Few Other Players

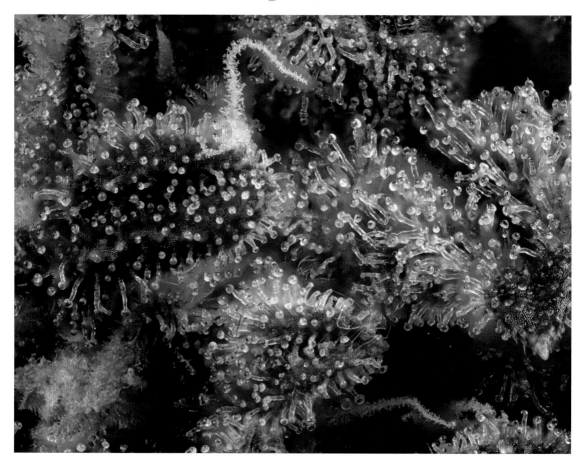

A macro detail of a cannabis bud with visible trichomes.

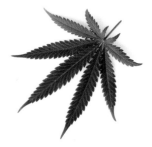

As mentioned, there are dozens—possibly upwards of a hundred—cannabinoids found in the marijuana plant. Some of these compounds haven't even been identified yet, and the restrictions on studying the plant have meant that discoveries have been slow. But scientists have isolated a few other cannabinoids and found that many of them have some unique benefits.

These are just a handful of the cannabinoids found in marijuana. With so many benefits already discovered, it seems logical that more research and study needs to be allowed on the marijuana plant. Who knows what other medicinal secrets could be unlocked?

Cannabigerol

Cannabigerol, or CBG, is one such compound. Like CBD, this compound is not psychoactive, but CBG is sort of a "stem cell" for other cannabinoids, and can eventually turn into THC or CBD. On its own, it has anti-anxiety and muscle relaxing effects, and studies have shown that it works as an anti-inflammatory.

Cannabichromene

Cannabichromene, or CBC, is another compound found in cannabis. It is also not psychoactive, making it another promising cannabinoid for the future of medicine. CBC is even better at treating anxiety than CBD, and the effects last longer because the compound stays in the bloodstream for a long time. It's also been found to be anti-inflammatory, anti-bacterial, and anti-fungal. Amazingly, a University of Mississippi study even discovered that CBC helped to promote brain growth.

Cannabinol

Another cannabinoid in marijuana is cannabinol, or CBN. Although CBN is not considered psychoactive, it can have a very strong sedative effect. CBN forms when THC reacts with oxygen, so the longer cannabis is exposed to air, the more CBN it will contain. Because of its ability to cause drowsiness, CBN shows promise for treating insomnia and nerve pain.

THCV

Similar to THC is the cannabinoid tetrahydrocannabivarin, or THCV. And just like THC, THCV is also psychoactive. But unlike THC, THCV actually suppresses appetite rather than stimulates it. Because of this property, THCV is being studied as a possible weight-loss drug. It's also been shown to reduce the tremors that result from Parkinson's disease.

A Plant by Any Other Name . . .

If you're new to the cannabis scene, you may assume that all marijuana is the same. But "marijuana" encompasses an entire world of different strains, which all come with their own pros and cons and affect users in different ways. Think of it like this: Chihuahuas, Huskies, and Rottweilers are all very different, but they have one thing in common: They're all dogs. But if you're looking for a dog that can comfortably nap on your lap while you watch TV, you probably won't choose a heavy Rottweiler; and if you need a good police dog, you probably won't go with a tiny Chihuahua!

Experts say that there are at least 779 strains of marijuana in the world, but that number continually changes because cannabis growers love to experiment with crossing different plants to create new hybrids. In fact, cannabis-friendly website Leafly.com lists more than 2,000 strains of marijuana! Amateur and professional growers alike love to give their new strains creative, colorful names like "Purple Urkle," "Frostbite," and "Liquid Butter." But all of the hundreds of varieties of marijuana in the world begin with three different species: *Cannabis indica*, *Cannabis sativa*, and *Cannabis ruderalis*.

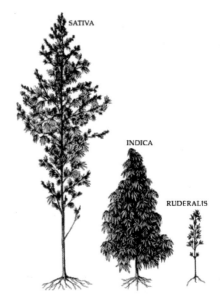

Cannabis was first identified as a monotypic species by eighteenth century botanist Carl Linnaeus. He classified the plant as *Cannabis sativa L.*, but in 1785, the botanist Jean-Baptiste de Lamarck identified a second species of cannabis, which he named *Cannabis indica*. One of the major differences between the species that Lamarck noticed was that the *sativa* species was better for producing strong fibers, while the *indica* species was better for inebriation.

Cannabis indica

Indica has traditionally been grown in parts of southeast Asia to produce *charas*, which is a type of hashish—the drug created from cannabis resin. The plant is short in stature, with broad leaves and a short flowering cycle, which makes it more ideal to colder climates with shorter growing seasons, or for indoor cultivation. Medicines produced with indica are said to induce mental and muscle relaxation, decrease nausea and pain, and increase appetite. The effects of indica are thought to be more sedating than other cannabis species, so many users consume the drug before bedtime or to relax at home. Some common indica strains include Northern Lights, Critical Mass, and L.A. Confidential.

Cannabis sativa

Sativa was first cultivated near the equator, in Thailand, Mexico, and Africa. The plant is tall, with narrow leaves and a long flowering cycle, and is often grown outdoors in warmer areas with longer growing seasons. Instead of producing a sedative effect, this species is said to energize users. It can reduce anxiety and depression, increase focus and creativity, and dull chronic pain. Because of its reputation for increasing energy, users often consume sativa in social situations or during creative pursuits. Some popular sativa strains include Durban Poison, Strawberry Cough, and Amnesia Haze.

Cannabis ruderalis

Ruderalis has traditionally been used in Russian and Mongolian folk medicine, and is thought to be especially useful for treating depression. On its own, this species is not psychoactive: ruderalis is naturally high in CBD and low in THC, so it's rarely grown for recreational use but prized for its medicinal properties. Ruderalis is a hardier plant than either indica or sativa, so it is able to resist disease and insects. It's also known for its very short growing season, and is mature in a matter of weeks. Because of these properties, ruderalis is often bred with indica or sativa to produce stronger, faster-growing plants with customized amounts of THC and CBD.

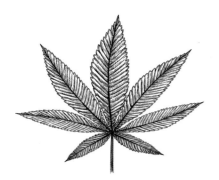

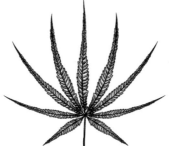

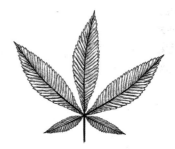

The leaves of *Cannabis indica* are much smaller than those found on plants of the *sativa* species. The leaflets are very wide without much separation between them. Usually there are about seven to nine leaflets on each leaf. The color of indica's leaves remains somewhat consistent with an olive green hue. Lighter shades of green are very rare and are usually a sign of a deficiency.

Cannabis sativa's leaves are larger than those of the *Cannabis indica* or *ruderalis* species. The separations between the leaflets can be very pronounced, and there can be up to thirteen leaflets on each leaf. The color of the leaves can range from bright or lime green to an almost blackish green.

Cannabis ruderalis' leaves can contain anything from five to thirteen leaflets, and they usually resemble the leaves of *Cannabis indica* more than those of *Cannabis sativa*, although the leaves of this species can be much narrower than you would normally find on an indica-dominant plant.

Does Species Matter?

Many cannabis users swear by these presumed indica/sativa differences when they choose a marijuana strain. Those who are looking to relax tend to choose indica; whereas those who want a pick-me-up go with sativa. But according to experts, these differences may not be standard across the board—with so many different strains to choose from, it stands to reason that not all indica strains will cause relaxation, and not all sativa strains will increase energy. So how can you choose a strain that will give you the effect you desire?

To That Effect

The effects of cannabis depend on a number of different things: the specific strain's chemical composition, your body chemistry and tolerance level, the dose, and the method of consumption. Perhaps the best indicator of what effects any given strain might have is the level of THC and CBD contained in each one. THC-dominant strains will have more of a potent effect and are more often chosen by those who seek relief from pain, depression, or insomnia. But THC-dominant strains can also cause unpleasant side effects—like anxiety, dry mouth, and red eyes—in some users. For those who are more sensitive to THC, a CBD-dominant strain may be best. These can help curb the side effects caused by THC, while still providing relief from symptoms like pain or depression. In fact, CBD works so well at counteracting THC's effects, that it can even be taken after using a THC-dominant strain if the strain is producing unwanted side effects.

Strains that balance THC and CBD make the most of this yin/yang effect, and many—especially novice users—find these to be the best choice for providing a desired outcome.

What's That Smell?

But there's another surprising attribute to consider when choosing a cannabis strain: terpenes. Terpenes are the aromatic compounds produced by flowers, plants, and fruit, and they are best known for being the basis for aromatherapy. If you've ever diffused a lavender oil to relax or felt energized by the scent of citrus, you understand the power of terpenes. The cannabis plant is the same way: different strains produce different scents, which in turn can provide users with uplifting or relaxing experiences.

Cannabis terpenes are produced in the same glands that produce the THC and CBD in the plant. More than a hundred of these aromatic compounds have been identified in cannabis, and depending on the strain, they can be scented like berries, citrus, spices, pine—or even cheese! Individual terpenes are associated with specific effects. It's a good idea to take a whiff of the strains you're thinking of using and see which ones appeal to you. In short, finding the right cannabis strain has less to do with indica versus sativa and more to do with what works for each individual.

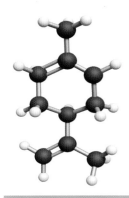

The terpene limonene elevates mood. It is the main constituent found in the oils of citrus peels and is commonly used for fragrances and food flavoring. It is also be used as a botanical insecticide, cleaning solvent, and paint stripper.

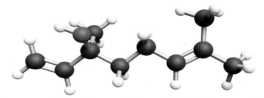

The terpene linalool has a relaxing effect like limonene. It is also used for its scent in products like shampoos, detergents, and soaps. Some insecticides used for cockroaches, fruit flies, and fleas contain linalool.

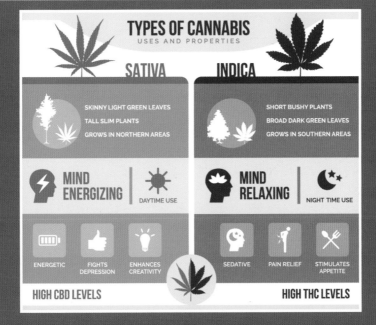

TYPES OF CANNABIS
USES AND PROPERTIES

SATIVA
- SKINNY LIGHT GREEN LEAVES
- TALL SLIM PLANTS
- GROWS IN NORTHERN AREAS

MIND ENERGIZING | DAYTIME USE

- ENERGETIC
- FIGHTS DEPRESSION
- ENHANCES CREATIVITY

HIGH CBD LEVELS

INDICA
- SHORT BUSHY PLANTS
- BROAD DARK GREEN LEAVES
- GROWS IN SOUTHERN AREAS

MIND RELAXING | NIGHT TIME USE

- SEDATIVE
- PAIN RELIEF
- STIMULATES APPETITE

HIGH THC LEVELS

Is There Really A Difference?

There is a lot of talk about the different effects each species, and even strains, produce. It is widely believed that indica-dominant strains will put you too sleep, while sativa-dominant strains will keep you energized and active. But that isn't necessarily the case, says Jeffery Raber, Ph.D., in a recent *LA Weekly* article. With a Ph.D. in chemistry, Raber might have some authority on the subject when he says that difference between sativa and indica strains "is just morphology"—meaning they just look different without being too different in terms of their chemical constituents. But what about the millions of joints that have been smoked in the name of research? It's hard to say what is true when the data of how the plant affects individual users is inherently subjective. Each user will be affected in different ways, and each plant has a variable potential to be more or less potent. One missing link in unlocking the difference between indica- and sativa-dominant strains might be the terpene profiles, which can give us a deeper genetic look into each plant, helping us understand each plant's characteristics, as opposed to categorizing the species as a whole.

Cultivating Cannabis

As we've seen, cannabis has been grown for millennia. At this point in history, humans are pretty much experts at cultivating marijuana and creating all kinds of inventive ways to use and consume it. Of course, it all starts with the plant itself.

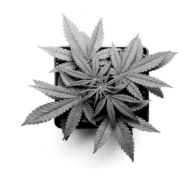

From Seed to Smoke

Cannabis can either be grown from a seed, or from stems taken from mature plants. Many professional growers prefer to use stems, to ensure their quality remains consistent. A cannabis plant grown from a stem will be a genetic replica of the original, so growers know exactly what to expect. After it's planted, the cannabis needs an optimal climate to thrive. The plant prefers to be warm (but not too warm!), growing well in temperatures between sixty-eight and seventy-seven degrees, and it likes humidity to be approximately sixty percent. Cannabis also likes a lot of light—when it's grown outdoors, cultivators find an area that receives at least twelve hours of sunlight a day. And when it's grown indoors, many experts prefer to keep artificial light on their plants twenty-four hours a day.

Professional growers also pay close attention to the nutrients they add to the soil and water, which is just another way they provide the plant with optimal growing conditions. When it's taken care of, cannabis grows quickly—a healthy plant can grow two inches in just one day! Once the plant reaches the flowering stage, it produces a sticky resin that coats the leaves—the resin contains the highest percentage of THC in the plant. The flowers—also called "buds"—are removed and hung to dry for a few weeks, and then they're ready to be consumed.

Marijuana is often called weed because of its ability to grow quickly and in a variety of situations. But to grow marijuana that is psychoactively and medicinally potent, you need to give the plant specific settings in which to grow. If done right, you can grow and cure your own marijuana within three to five months.

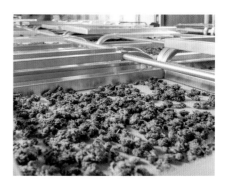

Curing buds can be as complicated or as easy as you want it to be. It all depends on how fast you expect your final product to be ready.

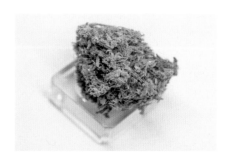

A cured bud ready for consumption.

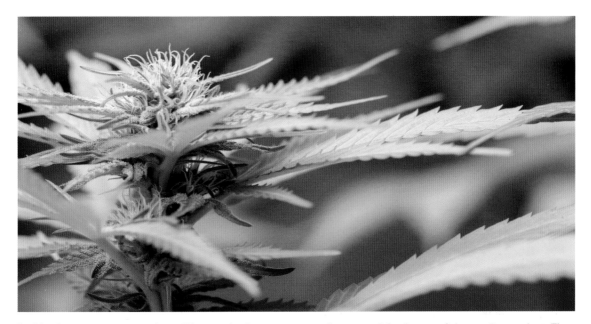

In this photo we can see a clear difference in the appearance of sugar and fan leaves of the marijuana plant. The fan leaves stretch far from the stem, while the sugar leaves are nestled much closer to the stem with resinous, white crystals collecting on them.

Two Types of Leaves

The buds are most commonly used for smoking, but they're not the only useful part of the plant. Cannabis plants also consist of two kinds of leaves: the fan leaves are the leaves that run along the length of the plant and have the characteristic shape common to marijuana, whereas the sugar leaves are the small leaves close to the bud that are covered in sugary resin. Most users don't smoke the leaves, because they contain fewer active ingredients than the buds. But this doesn't mean the leaves are useless! They can be baked into cookies or cakes, made into tea, or used for juicing.

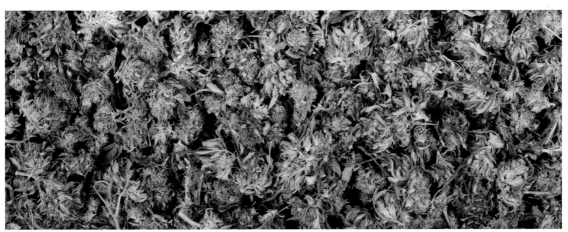

What Is Kief?

The shiny, sticky resin found on cannabis flowers is made up of trichomes. If you look really closely, these trichomes resemble tiny glass mushrooms, with a stalk and a bulbous head. That tiny bulbous part of the trichome contains the highest concentration of cannabinoids in the entire plant, and when it's collected, you have a concentrated form of cannabis known as kief.

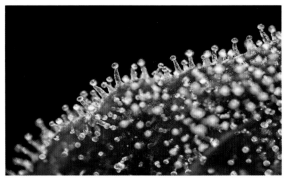

After a marijuana bud is cured and dried, the trichomes dry out as well and create a pollen-like substance known as kief. Kief is much more psychoactively potent than the dried buds of marijuana because it contains larger percentages of THC.

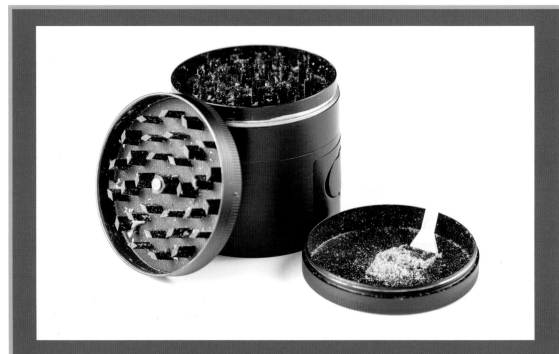

Collecting Kief

To separate the kief from the rest of the plant, many growers use old-fashioned elbow grease. A favorite method to ensure the purest product possible is to sift plant matter through smaller and smaller screens, until only the trichome bulbs remain. An easier method is to use a grinder with a mesh screen to break up the plant and catch the kief, but trichome stems and other plant matter can be mixed in with the final product. Pure kief is only the bulb of the trichome and nothing else, so it can take some work to make sure that there are no undesirable ingredients in the mix.

Consuming Kief

Once enough kief is collected, there are several ways it can be consumed. One of the easiest ways is to smoke it by sprinkling some onto a few buds and rolling it up. Kief can also be smoked on its own, but many users find it to be difficult because of kief's powdery consistency—rolling it with buds gives the substance something to stick to.

But for those who do want to smoke pure kief, it can be packed into a pipe. Since kief is much more potent than buds of marijuana, it's important to start conservatively with the amount—a little goes a long way! Vaporizers provide another way to consume the substance; and since some cannabinoids are immediately burned off when flame is applied to kief, they help preserve the THC and other beneficial ingredients. Vaporizers heat at a low enough temperature that none of the main components of the cannabis are destroyed.

Kief can also be used to make homemade e-cigarette cartridges by adding the substance to a 1:1 ratio of vegetable glycerin and propylene glycol and simmering in a double boiler. You can even add flavorings like berry or lemon if you'd like. Once the mixture has a smooth consistency, simply strain through a coffee filter and let it cool, then use a syringe to fill up your e-cigarette cartridge.

Cooking with kief is also a great way to use it, as it has a more subtle flavor than cannabis buds so it won't overpower the flavor of the finished recipe. It can be used on its own, or in combination with buds. But again, since kief is more potent than the buds, less can be used for the same effect.

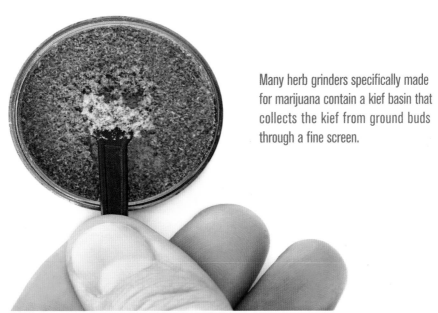

Many herb grinders specifically made for marijuana contain a kief basin that collects the kief from ground buds through a fine screen.

What Is Hash?

There's one more way that kief can be used: the substance can be used to make hash. Like kief, hash is composed of the bulbous part of cannabis trichomes; but to create hash, the kief must be heated and pressed to form a packed, solid brick. Pressing kief into hash is thought to have originated around 900 AD near Egypt, where the final product was called "hashish." Centuries later it made its way to Europe, where it became popular amongst the literary scene in Paris, and was consumed by writers like Victor Hugo, Alexandre Dumas, and Honore de Balzac.

By the late 1800s, hash was used medicinally in the U.S., where it was prescribed for pain, migraines, and insomnia, but eventually it fell out of favor as new medicines came on the market. During the 1900s, the drug was mostly found in Europe and Morocco—which is still a major hash producer—where it was used more often than herbal cannabis. Europeans still consume more hash than other forms of marijuana, but the substance is becoming more popular in the U.S. as cannabis restrictions are lifted and more and more people try their hand at home cultivation.

Hash: To Eat or to Smoke?

Traditionally, hash was consumed orally, either eaten as a solid or infused into drinks. In fact, Indians still drink a beverage called bhang, which is a milk-based drink mixed with spices and hashish. And American writer Fitz Hugh Ludlow wrote his most famous book, *The Hashish Eater*, to chronicle his own experiences with the drug. Nowadays, users often smoke the substance—sometimes mixed with regular tobacco.

Before trying any kind of hash product, it's important to remember that it's a very concentrated product compared to marijuana buds. Where even the strongest strains of marijuana buds clock in at around thirty percent THC, hash can have up to ninety percent THC content.

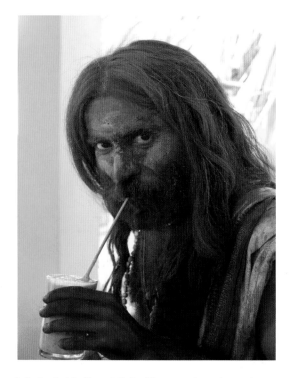

A spiritual teacher drinking bhang at a holy festival in Hampi, India. Marijuana is an integral part to some denominations of the Hindu religion. It is debated that marijuana is the plant identified as "soma" in the *Rigveda* and that it is also the favorite food of the Hindu god Shiva.

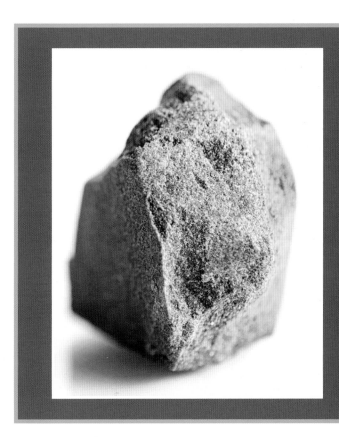

A Simple Process

Making hash from kief is a surprisingly simple process: A quick internet search gives users all the info they need to get started. One of the simplest ways to create a brick of hash is to place some kief between two pieces of parchment paper and then use a warm iron to press it all together. Just be sure not to let the paper burn!

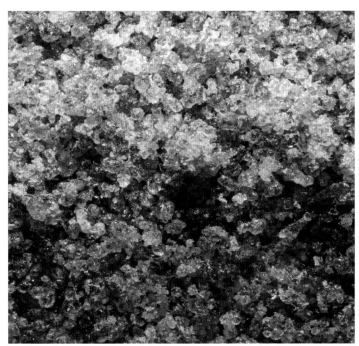

Hash can be made with a variety of processes. The water-purified process produces what is known as Bubble Hash. Separating the trichomes from the rest of the plant is the most labor intensive part of the process and can sometimes require the uses of solvents like ethanol, butane, or hexane.

No Smoking? No Problem!

If the thought of breathing in a cloud of smoke just isn't your thing, but you're still interested in experimenting with cannabis, you're in luck: Edible marijuana products are becoming more and more popular. Many users prefer this method of consumption because there is no telltale "marijuana" smell, no secondhand smoke to worry about, and it's convenient. What's more, when cannabis is eaten, the effects last longer, which can be a huge positive for those who use the drug for relief from pain or anxiety.

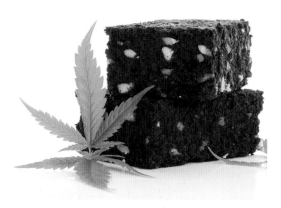

We've all seen a movie or television show where a character accidentally ingests some pot brownies and hilarity ensues. But today's edibles go way beyond baked goods—nowadays, you can find cannabis in everything from soft drinks to beef jerky to gourmet truffles. However, to pack these foods with the right amount of punch, it takes more than just mixing in a few marijuana buds. Cannabis must first undergo a process called decarboxylation before the THC within the plant can cause any effects.

Decarboxylation

In its natural state, cannabis is actually non-psychoactive—if you were to munch on a few raw cannabis leaves or flowers, you wouldn't feel the "high" associated with marijuana. This is because when it's live and growing, the plant is full of a cannabinoid called tetrahydrocannabinolic acid, or THCA. And while THCA has been found to have many of the same medicinal properties as other cannabinoids, it does not create any psychoactive effect. But after cannabis flowers have been collected and dried, the "acid" in THCA begins to break down and the compound starts to convert into THC. To speed up this conversion, heat can be used—this is decarboxylation.

When cannabis is smoked, the decarboxylation is instantaneous, because flame is applied directly to it—basically, the heat "activates" the THC in the plant. So to enjoy marijuana's effects in edible form, the cannabis used in each recipe must first undergo decarboxylation. THC easily binds with fats, so many people like to heat butter or oils with cannabis to unlock the THC and infuse the ingredients with cannabinoids. The butter or oil can then be mixed into whatever recipe is desired. Homemade "cannabutter" recipes can be found online, so bakers can create their own cannabis cookies, cakes, or yes, even the ubiquitous brownies.

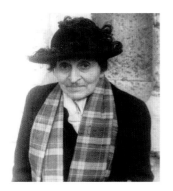

Alice B. Tolkas, life partner of writer Gertrude Stein, is considered to have published the first modern culinary recipe to call for the use of cannabis. Her book, *The Alice B. Toklas Cookbook*, described a Hashish Fudge that included spices, nuts, and fruits. The fudge was guaranteed to enliven any social gathering with the onset of fits of laughter and floods of thought. The recipe was supposedly given to her by Brion Gysin, a good friend of William S. Burroughs, and Toklas even goes so far as to suggest where her readers might acquire some cannabis.

Be Patient, Use Caution

One thing to remember with edibles: It takes longer for the cannabis to take effect, because unlike smoking the drug—which is absorbed by the lungs—edibles find their way into the bloodstream and are absorbed by the liver. The process can take an hour or two, so it's important to let the effects take hold before consuming too many cannabis-infused edibles. Drinks provide a way to avoid this problem, because they are sublingual—meaning absorption starts in the mouth—so effects take hold within five to thirty minutes.

Another edible option is dissolvable cannabinoid powders. These powders have very little taste or smell, which means they can not only be added to your favorite teas, drinks, and smoothies, but can be added to just about any recipe you can think of. They give a whole new meaning to the phrase "secret ingredient"!

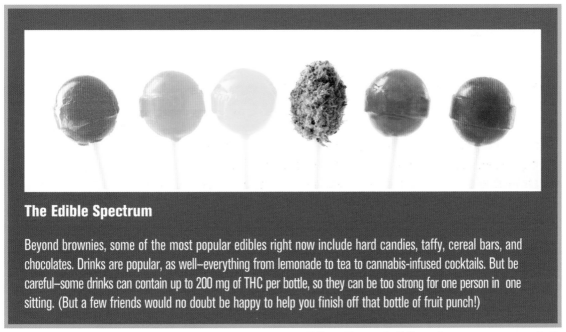

The Edible Spectrum

Beyond brownies, some of the most popular edibles right now include hard candies, taffy, cereal bars, and chocolates. Drinks are popular, as well—everything from lemonade to tea to cannabis-infused cocktails. But be careful—some drinks can contain up to 200 mg of THC per bottle, so they can be too strong for one person in one sitting. (But a few friends would no doubt be happy to help you finish off that bottle of fruit punch!)

Oils, Waxes & Concentrates

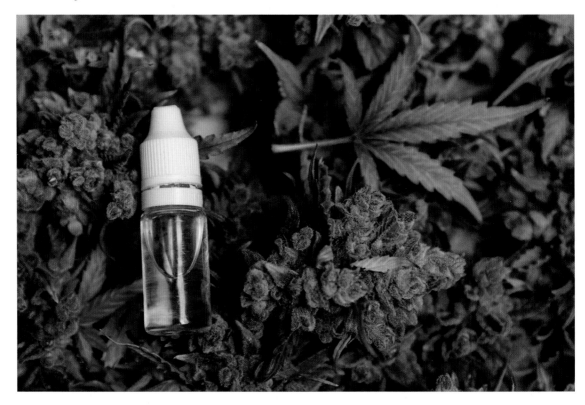

Before cannabis was labeled an illegal drug, it was extremely common for people to have the drug in their home medicine cabinets. In fact, prior to the Marijuana Tax Act of 1937, the most common way to consume cannabis was in the form of tinctures. Today, tinctures—and other forms of cannabis concentrates—are making a comeback, thanks to their ease of use and convenience. Technically, kief and hash are concentrates, as they make use of only the highly potent resin glands of the cannabis trichomes; but there are plenty of other cannabis concentrates to choose from.

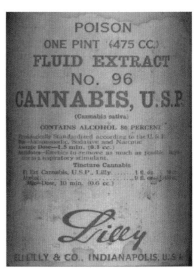

Marijuana was accepted into the United States' pharmacopeia in 1850 with medical benefits for various diseases like neuralgia, tetanus, typhus, cholera, rabies, dysentery, alcoholism, opioid addiction, insanity, leprosy, incontinence, snakebites, gout, tonsillitis. Companies like Eli Lilly & Co. were able to sell tinctures like this in pharmacies and grocery stores.

Oils

Cannabis oils are one such choice. The oils are made by using alcohol, olive oil, or CO_2 to extract cannabinoid resin. The finished product is extremely high in cannabinoids, so only a small amount is needed to produce an effect. The most popular oils are CBD oil and THC oil. The main difference, of course, is that CBD oil causes no psychoactive effects, so it can be used at any time during the day without interrupting your usual routine. But used medicinally, these two different oils also each have their place when treating different ailments.

CBD oil is extremely popular right now, especially because most states have legalized the substance, and it can easily be purchased online. But do your research before buying: Some online retailers only offer "hemp" oil, which is generally extracted from the seeds of the cannabis plant and contains very little CBD. True CBD oil is extracted from the leaves, flowers, and stems of the plant, and results in a much higher percentage of CBD. The oil has anti-inflammatory properties, which makes it good for treating joint pain and arthritis, and it helps to relieve anxiety and depression. There have also been very promising studies of CBD oil's effects on neurological disorders like epilepsy and Parkinson's disease.

THC oil is often used to stave off nausea and vomiting in chemotherapy patients. And thanks to THC's penchant for causing "the munchies," it can also increase appetite and help patients gain weight. The oil is also prized for its pain-relieving properties. But some of the best effects may come from combining CBD oil with THC oil. For instance, studies have shown that multiple sclerosis patients who take both CBD and THC oils can reduce muscle spasms by seventy-five percent. And cancer patients who receive CBD and THC report a significant reduction in pain compared to THC alone.

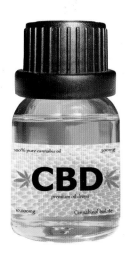

In 2018, the United States began allowing the sale of food and drink products containing CDB, but studies have found that many products purportedly containing CBD do not. It is best to do your research into a product to ensure that it contains what it says it does.

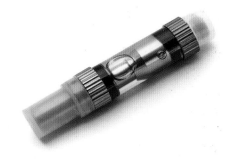

THC oil is a very concentrated form of the marijuana plant's most psychoactive properties, consisting of up to eighty to nearly ninety-nine percent THC. Usually one pound of dried marijuana will produce one tenth to one fifth of that in THC oil after the extraction process.

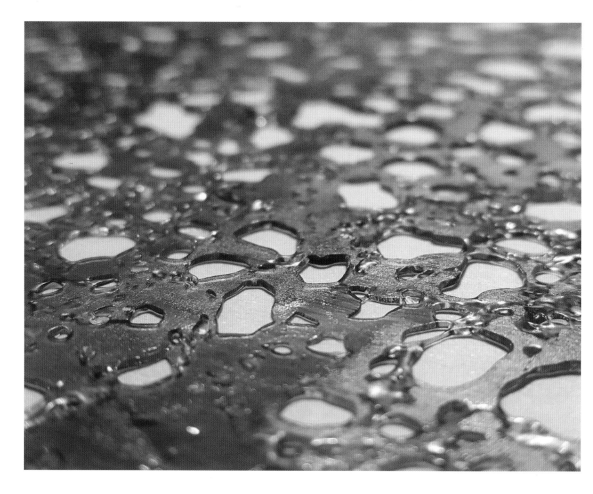

Oils, waxes, and concentrates are all extracted from the marijuana plant with processes that require butane, CO_2, or hydrocarbon. These solvents are not considered to be harmful because they evaporate during the processing of the concentrates. Shatter, seen here, is considered one of the most potent marijuana products available today.

Waxes

Another concentrated form of cannabis is wax, which is also known as butane hash oil. As the name suggests, this wax is derived by packing buds of marijuana in a tube and blasting it with butane—a highly flammable substance. The process can be dangerous, so experimenting with homemade cannabis wax is definitely not recommended: Leave it to the experts! The extraction process either leaves behind a crumbly, sticky substance—called "honeycomb"—or a harder, glasslike substance—known as "shatter." The extremely potent wax is most commonly used with vaporization methods, and is popular for treating chronic pain.

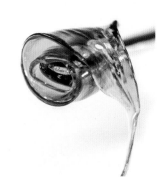

Sometimes called Green or Golden Dragon, THC and CBD tinctures are often considered much stronger than they actually are because of their intimidating street names. Tinctures are a good way for newcomers to the marijuana world to test the water with controlled dosages. Tinctures can easily be measured and added to a variety of foods and drinks for consumption.

Tinctures

The tinctures of old are slowly finding their way back into modern-day medicine cabinets. Basically, tinctures are cannabis-infused alcohol, and they can easily be made at home with a few simple ingredients. One of the great features of tinctures is that they can be stored for years in a cool, dry place, without losing potency. They're also simple to measure out, so once you find your desired dosage, you can easily consume the perfect amount without worrying about too little or too much of an effect. Tinctures can also be added to drinks, soups, smoothies, salad dressings, or even ice cream. But if you'd rather forego the food and still have a palatable concentrate, flavorings can be added. If the tincture is added to food and consumed, the effects are much like other edibles—the cannabis must make its way to the liver and it can take up to two hours for the effects to kick in. But placed under the tongue and held in the mouth for about thirty seconds, tinctures are immediately absorbed by the arterial blood supply and effects can be felt in fifteen to forty-five minutes. For someone using the remedy for pain relief, the faster the effect, the better.

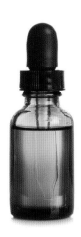

Balms

What if you want to experience some of marijuana's benefits, but don't care for a "high" feeling or any other intoxicating side effects? Topicals may be just the thing you're looking for. Used mainly for relief of pain, soreness, and inflammation, topical cannabis products come in the form of lotions, balms, sprays, and oils that are rubbed into the skin. They may seem like a brand new way to enjoy cannabis, but there's evidence that Egyptians and Africans used cannabis topically thousands of years ago!

CB2 Binding

Manufacturers of topicals try to maintain the specific cannabinoids and terpenes found in whichever strain of marijuana they use for their balms and lotions. They may also mix in essential oils or other therapeutic ingredients like cayenne, wintergreen, or lavender. The active ingredients work by binding to CB2 receptors in the body; but since the ingredients don't make their way to the bloodstream, they can't produce any psychoactive effects. (The exception would be transdermal patches, which are quickly making their way into the cannabis market. These patches do deliver cannabinoids into the bloodstream, so if they contain a high THC content, they can produce a "high.")

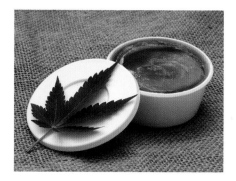

Balms have become very popular among athletes and people who suffer from joint or chronic pain.

Topicals are already a popular choice for localized pain relief and muscle soreness, but as more users discover their benefits, anecdotal evidence suggests that the products could also help to quell psoriasis, itching, cramps, and headaches. The added ingredients in topicals can work with the cannabinoids to increase their effectiveness. For instance, if you're looking to soothe muscles after a hard workout, try a balm with peppermint or wintergreen. For more localized pain relief, look for a warming lotion with cayenne.

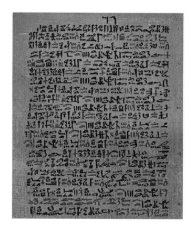

The Ebers papyrus is a medical document recording the herbal knowledge of ancient Egypt dating from circa 1550 BC. Although it has many hundreds of magical rituals and incantations used for remedies, it does show that there was a long history of the empirical study of medicine in ancient Egypt. The Ebers papyrus contains a prescription to treat inflammation by applying marijuana directly to the skin.

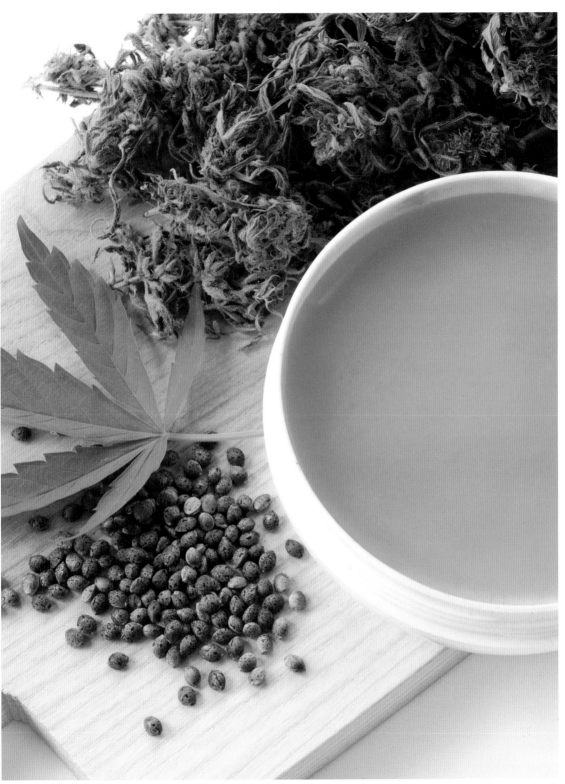

It Goes Where?

We've seen a huge variety of cannabis products and a multitude of ways to use them. In fact, it might seem as if we've exhausted all the marijuana choices on the market; however, there's still one more way to consume cannabis: in the form of a suppository. And yes, we are, in fact, talking about that kind of suppository. They may not often be discussed by most marijuana mavens, but cannabis suppositories, which can be placed either in the rectum or vagina, have some surprising advantages.

Discussing suppositories no doubt induces a few uneasy giggles, but the origins of this unusual delivery method are quite serious. As the popularity of medicinal cannabis has grown, more and more people suffering from pain and serious illnesses have turned to the plant in a desperate search for a medicine that works. Many have found that cannabis is just the remedy they're looking for—but not everyone is able to handle the psychoactive effects of products with high THC amounts.

To help these patients, caregivers discovered that administering high-THC cannabis in suppository form was the perfect answer. When administered in this way, the cannabis is still absorbed into the bloodstream; but since it bypasses the liver, it doesn't result in a psychoactive "high." Users get all the benefits of THC but remain clear-headed. The method is also good for those who have trouble swallowing due to severe nausea or vomiting, or for terminally ill patients.

Fast Acting Alternative

Avoiding a "high" isn't the only advantage of the suppository method. For example, inhaling or ingesting marijuana can lower its effectiveness so that only twenty percent of available cannabinoids are used by the body. But suppositories consistently deliver fifty to seventy percent of the plant's therapeutic properties. This method is also fast acting: Effects can be felt within fifteen minutes, and they last for four to eight hours.

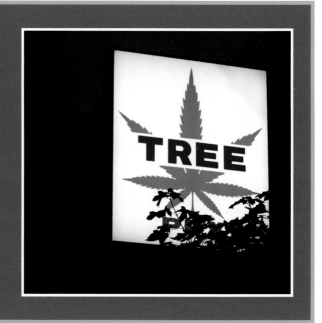

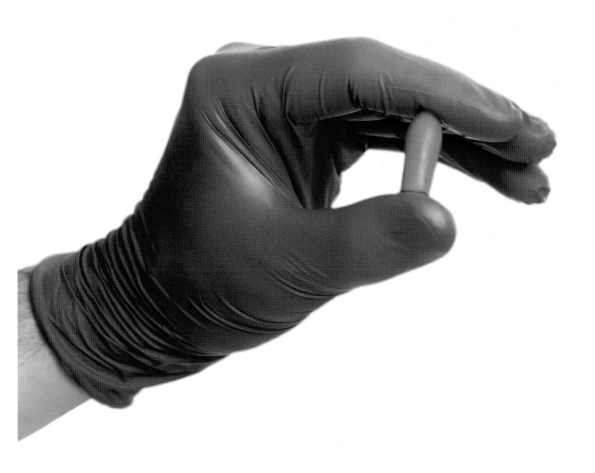

Cannabis in suppository form can be harder to find than other consumption methods, especially in states that are new to the legal marijuana scene. But it may be worth the search to find them, if the psychoactive side effects of cannabis are too much to bear.

Chapter 3

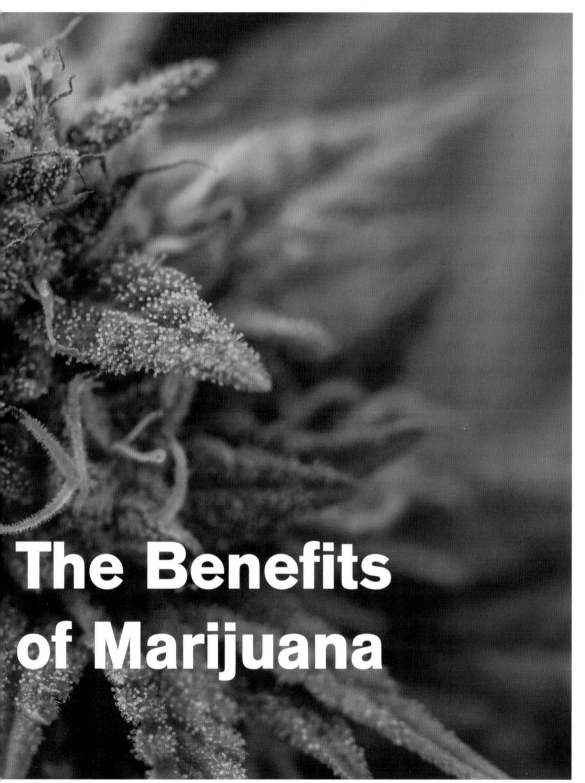

The Benefits of Marijuana

The Pain Process

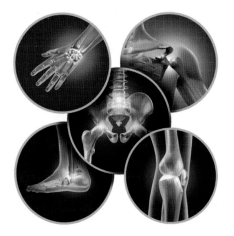

The world of cannabis is surprisingly diverse. With upwards of two thousand different strains and a myriad of products created from them, there's something in the mix for everyone. And that's great news, because those who suffer from a multitude of ailments and disorders—people from all walks of life—may find the relief they need in this amazing plant. Wondering what sorts of symptoms may benefit from medicinal cannabis? Let's start from the beginning.

The Mechanics of Pain

Pain may be the most basic and ubiquitous malady affecting humans. We've all felt it—everything from a tiny splinter under the skin to a broken bone can cause unpleasant, or even unbearable, sensations. Pain can be sharp, burning, dull, or achy—the pain we feel from a headache is different from the pain we feel from a sunburn. If the onset is sudden and lasts only a short amount of time, it is acute pain; but if it is unrelenting and lasts for months—or longer—it is chronic pain. As upsetting as pain is, it has an important function: mainly, to alert you of a dangerous situation within your body. The nerve cells that produce pain are part of the peripheral nervous system—this includes all of the body's nerves except those in the spine and brain, which make up the central nervous system. When nerve endings are stimulated—such as when you stub your toe or cut yourself—special peripheral nerve cells called "nociceptors" send a pain message in the form of electrical impulses to the brain.

The International Association for the Study of Pain originally classified pain with five criteria: 1) where on the body it occurs, 2) anatomical system causing the pain, 3) duration and pattern of pain, 4) intensity, and 5) cause. However this type of classification has come under some scrutiny from Harvard Medical School neurobiologist Clifford J. Woolf, who has created a new set of criteria for understanding pain. These criteria are 1) nociceptive pain, which is caused by stimulation of the sensory nerve fibers, 2) inflammatory pain associated with tissue and immune cell damages, and 3) pathological pain, which is caused by damage to the nervous system.

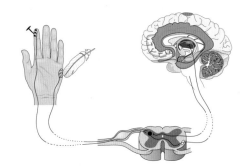

Painful stimulus in the hand sends information through afferent nerves that travel up the pathways along the spinal column and up to the thalamus. The thalamus consists of two different masses of gray matter that are positioned between the two cerebral hemispheres. The thalamus is responsible for pain perception and relaying sensory information.

The spinal cord actually sorts through the messages from these nociceptors to determine their urgency. Burning pain from a hot stove is deemed urgent, which then triggers your muscles to react by moving away from the source of the heat. But the pain from a mild scratch is relayed more slowly, resulting merely in a bit of discomfort. Once the pain messages reach the brain, the brain can send out its own messages, like signaling white blood cells to rush to an injury site, or flooding the body with pain-suppressing endorphins.

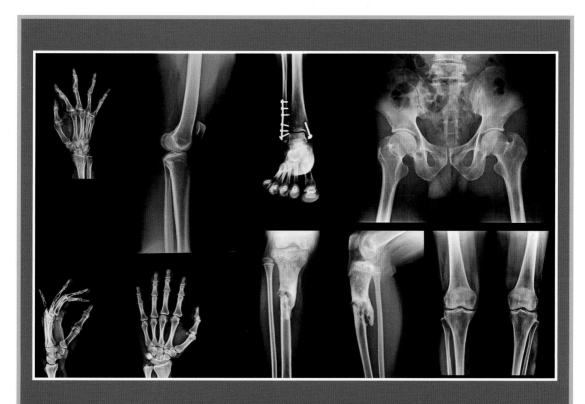

Perceiving Pain

How you ultimately perceive pain depends on several factors. Genetics play a role, not only with pain tolerance but also with how you respond to pain medications. Psychological factors can come into play as well—those who suffer from depression and anxiety tend to feel more pain than those who don't. And even having a pessimistic attitude toward pain can make it feel worse! Past experiences can also influence how pain is perceived: If you've already had a painful past experience with a situation—say, at the dentist—your body is more likely to produce a pain response during subsequent scenarios. Interestingly, the biggest risk factor for developing a painful condition is having already experienced a painful condition.

Treating Pain

It's obvious that pain is a complex process, and certainly one we'd all prefer to avoid. So when patients are overwhelmed with unrelenting pain, they're grateful to try any treatments their doctors may offer. Many times, that treatment plan includes opioid pain medications such as hydrocodone, fentanyl, and morphine. These narcotics work by binding to receptors in the brain and blocking all those pain messages sent by the peripheral nervous system. They're sort of like bouncers standing outside a nightclub—pain may be all dressed up, but because an opioid is standing in front of the velvet rope, it has nowhere to go.

Opioids can be very effective at managing chronic pain, but they come with some serious drawbacks. They can be highly addictive, especially when needed for long-term pain. And once use is discontinued, they can cause uncomfortable withdrawal symptoms like insomnia, vomiting, muscle and bone pain, and chills. But even worse than addiction and withdrawal is the possibility of overdose: When taken in large doses, or combined with other medications or alcohol, opioids can cause users to stop breathing. And frighteningly, this scenario plays out nearly 175 times a day in the United States.

The molecular structure of morphine.

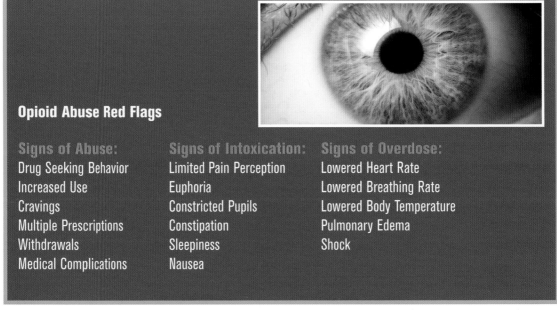

Opioid Abuse Red Flags

Signs of Abuse:	Signs of Intoxication:	Signs of Overdose:
Drug Seeking Behavior	Limited Pain Perception	Lowered Heart Rate
Increased Use	Euphoria	Lowered Breathing Rate
Cravings	Constricted Pupils	Lowered Body Temperature
Multiple Prescriptions	Constipation	Pulmonary Edema
Withdrawals	Sleepiness	Shock
Medical Complications	Nausea	

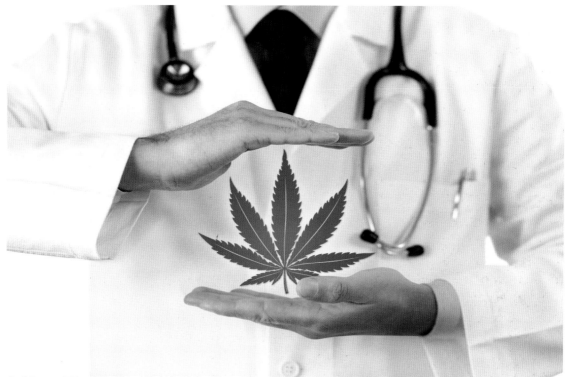

A New Method

But what if there was another way to treat chronic pain without these risks? This is where marijuana steps in. When someone uses marijuana, the drug can help dull pain in a few ways. Both THC and CBD have been shown to decrease inflammation, which can reduce pain at the site of injuries. THC can control pain by binding with CB1 receptors in the brain, and CBD can actually dampen pain signals as they make their way into the brain.

Unfortunately, those using cannabis for pain can develop a tolerance to it, so more and more is needed to produce the same effect. But the good news is, it's incredibly difficult to overdose on cannabis, as the amount needed to produce toxic effects is more than anyone could realistically consume. And more good news: to "reset" the brain back to its normal setting and reduce the amount of marijuana needed, a user only needs to take a short break from the drug. Studies show that the brain begins to return to normal after only two days of abstinence, and is fully back to normal after about four weeks.

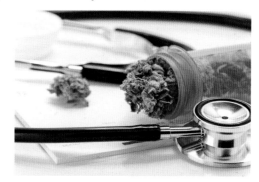

There are no serious adverse effects tied to the consumption of medical marijuana. Some may be negatively affected by nausea, tiredness, dizziness, and increased appetite, but the effects become much more tolerable after just a few uses.

An Answer

Reducing overdoses is just one benefit of treating pain with marijuana instead of opioids. Opioids, for instance, can cause cognitive impairment, to the point that those who are using them for severe pain may not even be able to communicate and function. But doctors have found that switching these patients over to cannabis has not only eased their pain, but also allowed them to effectively interact with their friends and family.

And while some people can develop a mild dependence on marijuana, the addiction is nowhere near as difficult to overcome as opioid dependence. Usually, a user who has become dependent on cannabis needs only behavior modification therapy and abstinence to break the habit, without the terrible withdrawal symptoms common to opioids.

Looking at the Numbers

Clearly, medicinal marijuana shows promise at being a safe, effective choice for pain, and studies are already proving it. In one study published in June 2017 in the journal *Cannabis and Cannabinoid Research*, almost three thousand patients who used opioids and cannabis to control their pain were surveyed. Of those patients, ninety-seven percent reported that cannabis allowed them to decrease their opioid use. And eighty-one percent felt that cannabis alone was even more effective than cannabis combined with opioids.

The stats coming out of states with legalized medicinal marijuana are encouraging, as well. Opioid use has already dropped in these areas—by as much as fourteen percent—as more and more people choose to bypass the drugs altogether and substitute cannabis. The relief found in this plant is so great that people suffering from pain have left their homes and made moves to states where cannabis is legal, just to avoid an opioid prescription. And recently, a small study suggested that the CBD in marijuana helps to reduce cravings of heroin addicts. So not only does cannabis replace opioids, but it may actually help people break their addictions to opioids!

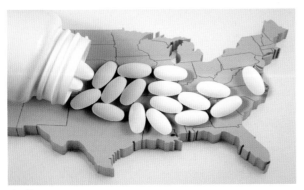

The problem with prescription opioids doesn't end with the pharmacy. If patients lose their prescriptions and have formed a dependence to the substance, they are much more likely to turn to illegal forms of pain killers like heroin.

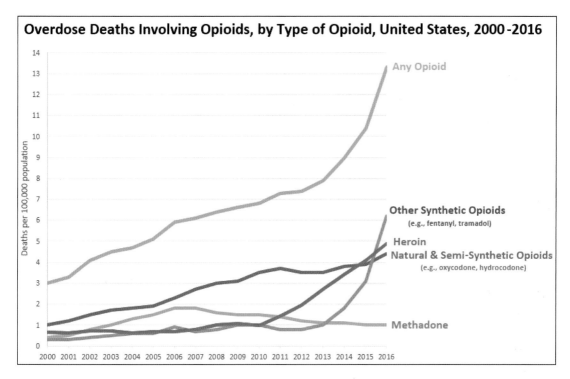

Overdose Deaths Involving Opioids, by Type of Opioid, United States, 2000-2016

Deaths per 100,000 population

- Any Opioid
- Other Synthetic Opioids (e.g., fentanyl, tramadol)
- Heroin
- Natural & Semi-Synthetic Opioids (e.g., oxycodone, hydrocodone)
- Methadone

Statistics of opioid deaths in the United States from the Centers for Disease Control and Prevention.

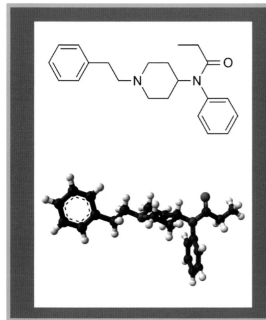

The Dangers of Fentanyl

Fentanyl is a very dangerous opioid that has become synonymous with the opioid epidemic in the U.S., Canada, and U.K. It is considered to be one hundred times stronger than morphine, with some of its analogues being nearly ten thousand times stronger than morphine. In British Columbia, according to the Coroner's Service, there were two overdoses a day throughout 2016—that number rose one-hundred percent the next year between January and April, with 368 deaths within that period. According to *The New York Times*, there were 21,000 deaths in the U.S. during 2016. Musicians Prince and Tom Petty both died of fentanyl overdoses.

Choosing a Remedy

Once you've decided to try treating your pain with cannabis, finding the right method isn't as easy as rolling a joint and puffing away. As with any medication, dosage and monitoring for side effects are both very important. And with thousands of strains of cannabis to choose from, finding the one that's right for you can take a bit of trial and error—a strain that causes one person to feel anxious might cause another to feel relaxed. So whatever strain you choose, always start with a small dose to see how it affects you. It's also advisable to choose something with a high CBD content—a 1:1 ratio of CBD to THC is a good place to start—because of CBD's anti-inflammatory effects and ability to mitigate some of the THC's intoxication.

The most popular methods used for those trying to relieve pain are vaporizing and edibles. It's suggested that first-time vapers take one hit and wait twenty minutes to see how they feel—if the pain continues and the psychoactive effects aren't prominent, another hit can be taken. For edibles, it's recommended to consume only a small amount of cannabis-infused food—amounting to about three mg of THC. And remember that the effects of edibles take longer to manifest, can be more potent than vaping, and can last longer.

While pain may be one of the most common reasons people seek out medicinal marijuana, it is by no means the only one. Cannabis shows promise for treating a host of different ailments, providing hope to suffering individuals. Let's take a look at some of the ways this plant is reshaping the future of medicine.

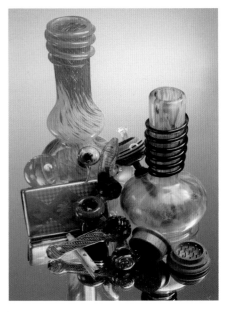

The paraphernalia you can use to smoke marijuana is vast. It may take a period of trial and error to find the right method.

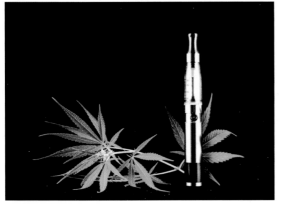

Vaporizers can be a very clean way to ingest marijuana, unlike smoking which can expose you to harmful carcinogens.

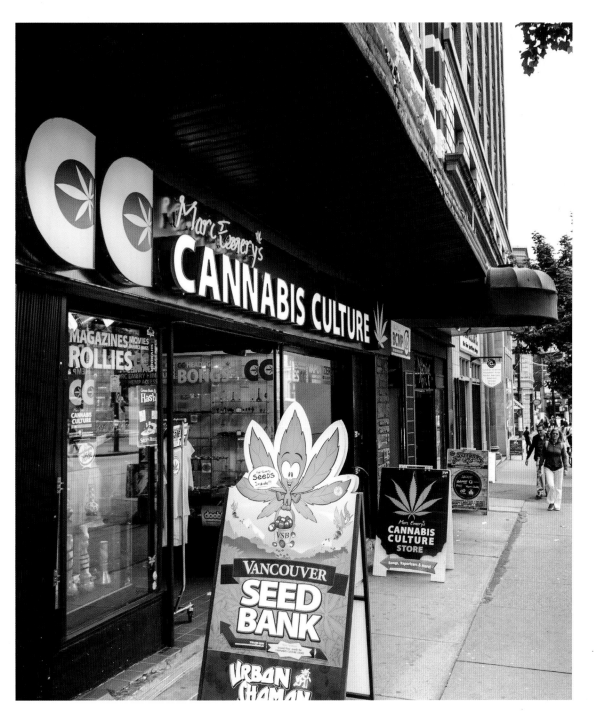

Your local smoke shop, or head shop, might be a good resource for you to begin with to find what method of ingesting marijuana is best for you.

Glaucoma

Normal vision

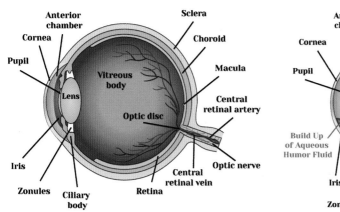

Glaucoma

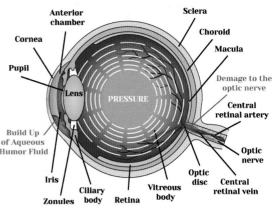

According to the magazine *Primary Care*, almost 67 million people in the world have glaucoma. There are 2 million people with glaucoma in the U.S.

Glaucoma is a relatively common condition which can affect everyone from babies to the elderly, although risk rises with age. In this eye disorder, fluid which normally flows in and out of the anterior chamber—a space at the front of the eye—drains out too slowly, causing a build-up of fluid and pressure. Over time, this pressure can damage the optic nerve, eventually leading to vision loss. Glaucoma accounts for approximately ten percent of all blindness in the U.S., and is the second-leading cause of blindness in the world. Most cases have no known cause, but occasionally tumors, diabetes, or advanced cataracts can bring on the condition.

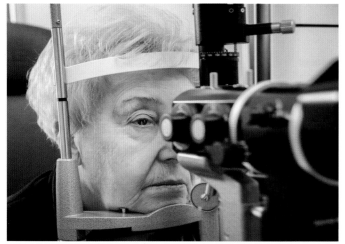

The causes of glaucoma are still somewhat unclear. Genetics, ethnicity, and inflammation can be factors. Prolonged steroid use and diabetic retinopathy are also factors that should be taken into account.

Treating Glaucoma

Treatments for glaucoma attempt to either improve the flow of fluid in the eye, or decrease its production. The first line of defense is usually eyedrops, which can result in various side effects. These can be as benign as stinging and redness, or as serious as retinal detachment and difficulty breathing. If the drops don't do the job, an oral medication that inhibits fluid production can be prescribed. If neither of these options works, surgery may be performed to reduce the pressure in the eye. This can involve using a laser to open clogged drainage canals in the eye, or implanting a silicone tube to increase drainage.

Unfortunately, none of these are a cure for glaucoma—they just help to keep symptoms under control. And in the 1970s, research began to show that marijuana was able to do likewise—the drug helped to lower pressure in the eye, temporarily keeping the disease's symptoms at bay. There is a drawback, however: Cannabis only lowers the pressure in the eye for a few hours, so a patient would need to consume marijuana throughout the day in order to treat the condition with cannabis alone. However, studies show that a combination of traditional treatment along with medicinal marijuana can be effective for some patients. Scientists are also working on creating THC eyedrops, which could deliver the benefits of the cannabinoid directly to the eye without THC's psychoactive side effects.

While it may not be ideal for most cases of glaucoma, medicinal cannabis is quite useful in later stages of the disease, when patients often suffer from nausea, vomiting, and anxiety. Cannabis is a great choice for treating these upsetting glaucoma side effects.

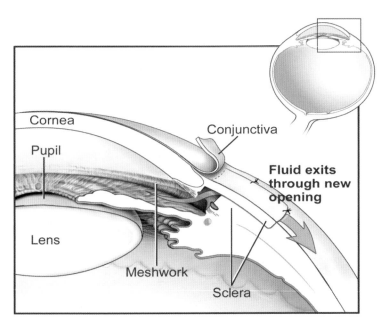

Surgery that has been conventionally used to treat glaucoma creates a new opening in the trabecular meshwork, which relieves pressure and provides a place for the excess fluid to drain from the eye.

Arthritis

When you hear the word arthritis, you may think of elderly people hobbling about, gripping canes with knobby fingers. But arthritis is actually a catch-all word that encompasses more than one hundred types of affliction, which can affect people of all ages. More than 50 million adults and 300,000 children have some type of the disease, which is the leading cause of disability in the U.S. Symptoms can include swelling, pain, and stiffness in one or more joints, and a decreased range of motion. Although the symptoms may come and go at first, over time, pain from arthritis can become chronic; this can make performing normal everyday tasks—like opening jars, climbing stairs, or even walking—difficult and uncomfortable.

Osteoarthritis

The most common type of arthritis is osteoarthritis. In this degenerative disease, the cartilage between bones wears away, until bone rubs on bone. Popular treatments include over-the-counter pain relievers, as well as using hot and cold compresses and engaging in regular exercise to strengthen the muscles surrounding the joint.

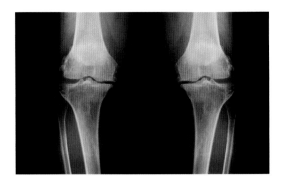

Inflammatory Arthritis

Inflammatory arthritis occurs when the immune system goes awry and begins attacking joints, as well as internal organs, eyes, and other body parts. Types include rheumatoid arthritis and psoriatic arthritis, and it can be treated with disease-modifying antirheumatic drugs, or DMARDs. The goal with inflammatory arthritis is to catch it early and achieve remission, in order to prevent permanent joint damage.

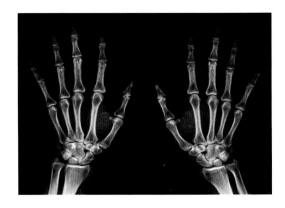

Other types of arthritis include infectious arthritis, which occurs when a bacteria, virus, or fungus causes joint inflammation, and metabolic arthritis—also called gout—which is caused by a buildup of uric acid in the body.

STAGE OF KNEE OSTEOARTHRITIS

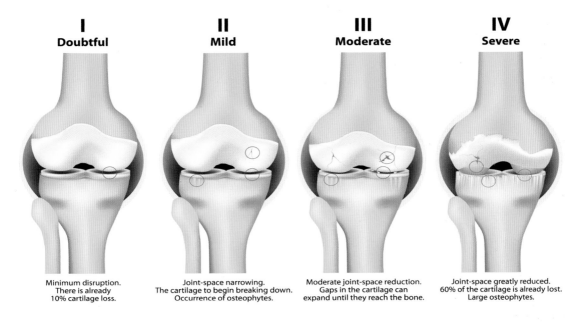

I Doubtful	**II** Mild	**III** Moderate	**IV** Severe

Minimum disruption. There is already 10% cartilage loss.

Joint-space narrowing. The cartilage to begin breaking down. Occurrence of osteophytes.

Moderate joint-space reduction. Gaps in the cartilage can expand until they reach the bone.

Joint-space greatly reduced. 60% of the cartilage is already lost. Large osteophytes.

According to the Centers for Disease Control and Prevention, women are more likely to suffer from arthritis than men. Old age also plays a role in the probability of being diagnosed with the disease.

How Marijuana Helps

Cannabis is becoming an increasingly popular remedy for all types of arthritis, due to its pain relieving and anti-inflammatory properties. What's more, researchers have discovered that the joints of arthritis sufferers contain an unusually high amount of CB2 receptors, making the drug an especially helpful choice for easing discomfort. And scientists are now conducting research to determine whether marijuana can not only relieve pain in the joints, but possibly repair damaged joints, as well.

Even mainstream medicine is starting to notice marijuana's effects on arthritis sufferers. And it's no wonder: THC has been found to have twice the anti-inflammatory power of hydrocortisone, and an impressive twenty times the power of aspirin! Those seeking relief from their arthritis symptoms often smoke or use vaporizers for their cannabis, but topicals are also a popular choice, as they can provide targeted relief to sore joints and muscles. And old-school tinctures are becoming more popular, especially for those who are new to medicinal marijuana.

Cancer

There are few words that sound as scary as *cancer*—hearing the diagnosis can be extremely frightening and overwhelming. For a disease that causes so much upheaval in people's lives, cancer is a surprisingly simple process: It occurs when cells in the body begin to grow out of control, crowding out normal cells and interrupting the usual functions of the body. Cancer cells can begin growing anywhere in the body, and then spread—or metastasize—to other areas.

In the United States, cancer is second only to heart disease in common causes of death. Over the last forty years, approximately $90 billion has been spent on cancer research and treatment, as scientists search for cures and ways to improve quality of life. And the good news is, deaths from cancer have been declining steadily for decades, falling twenty-six percent since 1991. Still, it is estimated that about 1.7 million Americans will be diagnosed with the disease this year, and approximately 600,000 will lose the battle.

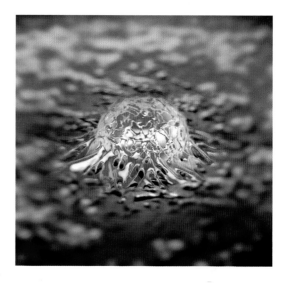

A photo of a breast cancer cell taken by a scanning electron microscope. There are several factors that contribute to a greater risk of developing breast cancer, including obesity, alcohol abuse, sedentary lifestyles, menstruating at a young age, child bearing at an old age, and a history of breast cancer in the family. The Cancer Institute claims that five to ten percent of breast cancer cases are inherited.

Traditional Treatments for Cancer

Such an insidious disease often requires aggressive treatment. Surgery can be used to remove as much cancer as possible, but often patients require chemotherapy or radiation treatments—or possibly both. Chemotherapy is a drug therapy that aims to kill cancer cells and prevent them from multiplying. Unfortunately, the treatment can inadvertently target healthy cells as well, leading to extreme side effects like nausea and vomiting, hair loss, fatigue, a loss of appetite, and depression. Radiation therapy, which targets cancer cells with high doses of radiation, can also cause similar unpleasant side effects.

The side effects of cancer treatment can be so bad that patients are unable to live normal lives. Some patients have described feeling nauseated all day, or feeling worse than with any bout of flu they've ever had. Weight loss is common, as it can be difficult to keep food down or to even have an appetite to begin with.

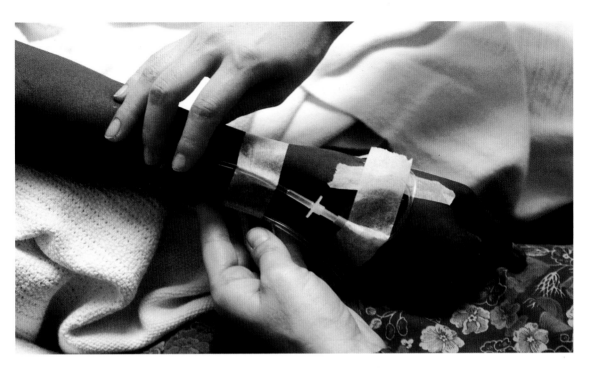

Chemotherapy therapy can be very effective for certain types of cancer. But not all types of cancer respond the way we want it to when treated with chemotherapy. It may be ineffective with brain tumors or not necessary with some types of skin cancer.

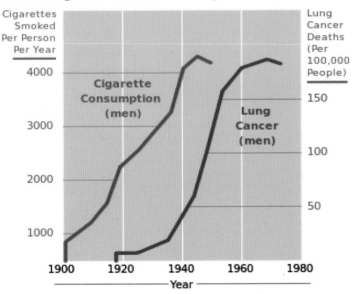

20-Year Lag Time Between Smoking and Lung Cancer

Inheriting cancer-causing genetics from your family line accounts for very few cases of cancer. According to a study from the National Center of Biotechnology Information, nearly ninety to ninety-five percent of cancer cases are caused by environmental factors causing genetic mutations. For example, the correlation between smoking tobacco and lung cancer is very high, as this chart from the National Cancer Institute shows. There are many dozens of carcinogens found in tobacco smoke including nitrosamines and polycyclic aromatic hydrocarbons.

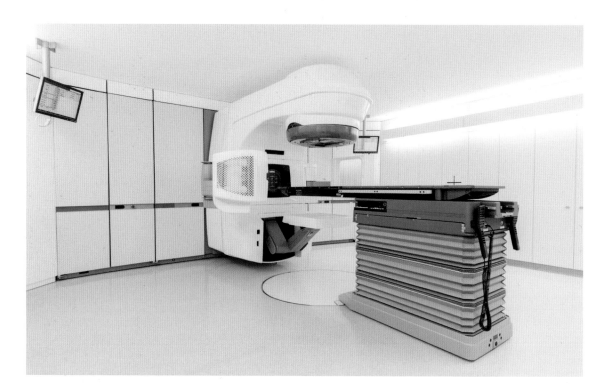

Radiation therapy for cancer can be very effective with cancers like leukemia and lymphoma. Unfortunately, there are many drawbacks to this type of treatment. For one, the larger the tumor the less the radiation has an effect in controlling the cancer. Also, there are a number of acute and long-lasting side effects that patients suffer from after treatment. Acute side effects include nausea, vomiting, mouth sores, swelling, infertility, and intestinal discomfort; while longer-lasting effects may cause cognitive decline, cancer, cardiovascular disease, fibrosis, and lymphedema.

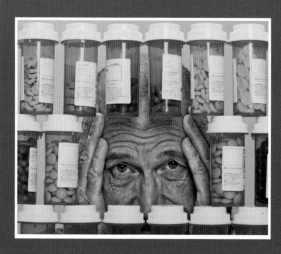

The Side Effects of Cancer Treatment

Cancer patients undergoing treatment might suffer from an array of side effects that might need prescription drugs to quell. These side effects include:

Anemia	Fertility Issues
Appetite Loss	Hair Loss
Delirium	Nausea
Diarrhea	Nerve Problems
Edema	Pain
Fatigue	Sleep Problems

How Can Marijuana Help?

Fortunately, those who live in states with medicinal marijuana laws have a reliable remedy to turn to: Marijuana has been repeatedly shown to be effective for calming nausea and vomiting in those undergoing chemotherapy or radiation. It also increases appetite, decreases anxiety, and prevents bouts of insomnia. In fact, sometimes cannabis is the *only* thing that brings these patients relief.

And there's another benefit to using cannabis when undergoing cancer treatment: Patients can often ditch a number of other prescriptions, thanks to marijuana's effects. When undergoing treatment, patients can be given up to a dozen different drugs to fight nausea, anxiety, headaches, and gastrointestinal problems. And all of those drugs can have their own side effects, as well—which adds up to a frustrating, and often ineffective, cocktail of pills. Grateful cancer patients have found that simply using cannabis—one single drug—can help quell their symptoms so well that they don't need a myriad of pills to function.

Best Practices for Ingestion

It is recommended that cancer sufferers try a vaporization method for cannabis, to ensure the effects are felt quickly—the sooner nausea is gone and appetite returns, the better! But to help ease symptoms overnight and prevent insomnia, patients can try an edible before retiring for the night—since the effects of edibles last longer, this can help guarantee a good night's sleep. There is also an FDA-approved drug called dronabinol, which is a synthetic form of THC and used to control nausea and vomiting and to increase appetite; however, since it is in pill form, it can be difficult for those suffering from severe nausea to swallow. Many patients prefer to stick with the real deal because dronabinol is lacking in all the other cannabinoids natural marijuana has to offer so.

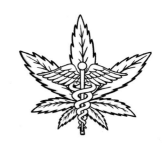

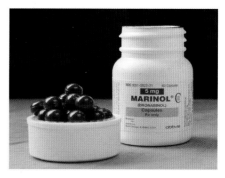

Marinol is the marketed brand name of dronabinol. Marinol was rescheduled from Schedule II to Schedule III of the Controlled Substance Act in 1999 after findings that THC had a lower risk of abuse than other substances in Schedules I or II.

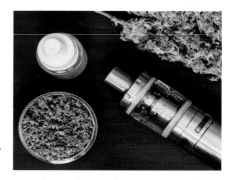

The Centers for Disease Control and Prevention states that it believes there is now sufficient evidence to say that vaping is less harmful than actually smoking, which can do wonders for someone who is undergoing cancer treatment.

Migraines

Headaches are one of the most common health issues in the world. They can be anywhere from annoying to downright debilitating. It's not uncommon for someone suffering from a painful headache to say they have a "migraine," but not all severe headaches are migraines—there are some marked differences between tension headaches and migraines that help doctors determine which a patient has.

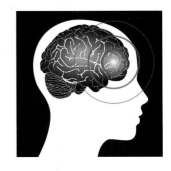

Differences Between Headaches and Migraines

Most headaches are tension headaches, which usually affect the whole head, and can feel like a band is wrapped around the skull. They can also affect the muscles of the neck and shoulders, causing aching and stiffness. The pain is usually mild to moderate—although it can occasionally be severe—and normally only last a few hours. Headache pain is generally a chronic, steady pain.

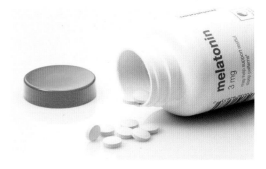

melatonin

A migraine, on the other hand, usually affects one side of the head, is moderately to severely painful, and has a throbbing quality that can be worsened by exertion. Migraines also are often accompanied by other symptoms called "auras," which can include nausea or vomiting, sensitivity to light, sound, or smells, vision changes, or numbness. Aura symptoms can occur ten to thirty minutes before the actual migraine hits. Some sufferers also experience subtle symptoms a day or two before getting a migraine, such as constipation, depression, irritability, or unusual mood changes.

Melatonin is a hormone produced in the pineal gland of animals and humans that helps with sleep regulation and wakefulness. Melatonin has begun to be accepted as a therapy for people to prevent migraines, although the evidence is not definitive.

Like tension headaches, migraines are first treated with over-the-counter medications like acetaminophen, aspirin, and ibuprofen. Some over-the-counter medications specifically marketed for migraines combine one or more of these drugs with caffeine, which helps the medication work more quickly. But when these remedies don't work, prescription drugs may be used to help the blood vessels around the brain contract and to increase serotonin levels in the brain. Anti-nausea drugs may also be prescribed. But when none of these options work, doctors may prescribe opioids like codeine or oxycodone.

Migraine Classification

Common migraines: pain without auras

Classic migraines: pain with auras

Retinal migraines: pain with visual distortions or temporary blindness

Probable migraines: pain with the characteristics of a migraine but without sufficient evidence to diagnose it as a migraine

Complications of migraine: pain and auras that are unusually frequent or too long (often associated with a brain lesion or seizure)

Chronic migraine: fulfills all of the criteria of a migraine headache and occurs very frequently, especially if the migraine reoccurs for fifteen days out of the month for three months

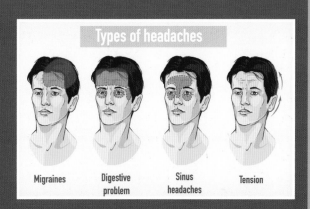

Types of headaches

Migraines   Digestive problem   Sinus headaches   Tension

How Marijuana Can Help

Fortunately, medicinal cannabis provides another option for those who suffer with this debilitating condition. And its effectiveness is backed up by more than just anecdotal evidence: a 2017 study showed that a combination of THC and CBD worked even better than prescription medication at staving off migraines, and the cannabinoids were able to cut migraine pain by forty-three percent. What's more, cannabis produced fewer unpleasant side effects than prescription medications. It seems that cannabis works so well because unlike prescription medications, it attacks the migraine from several different angles: pain, nausea, and inflammation.

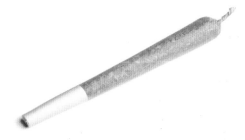

Inhalation methods are the most popular for easing migraine pain, as they provide the fastest relief. Rubbing a drop of oil into the gums or placing a drop of a tincture under the tongue can also provide quick relief. Edibles are less popular for migraine pain, as the effects can take up to two hours to manifest— and for a migraine sufferer, that's two hours too long!

Anorexia

It is far too easy for us to look into a mirror and pick out our flaws, but for someone suffering from anorexia, a distorted body image can lead to life-threatening consequences. Anorexia is characterized by severe calorie restriction, difficulty gaining weight, and compulsive exercising. Those who have this disorder may also lose interest in activities most people find enjoyable, resulting in isolation from friends and social activities.

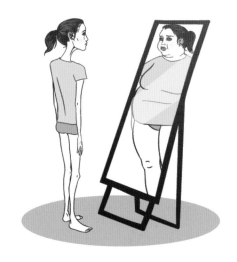

The disorder can affect people of ages and genders, and not all who suffer with anorexia are underweight—it's possible to be a normal weight, or even overweight, and still have the disorder. Anorexia can also affect patients with cancer or HIV/AIDS, as a side effect of illness or treatments. But as a psychiatric disease, anorexia has a frightening mortality rate: nearly thirteen percent of sufferers succumb to this disorder, the highest mortality rate of any mental illness.

Surprisingly, anorexia is highly heritable from family members. A person who has immediate family members who are anorexic is nearly twelve times more likely to develop anorexia. A 2011 study published in *Behavioral Neurobiology of Eating* states that the heritable risk of anorexia is twenty-eight to fifty-eight percent.

Treating Anorexia

Treatment for anorexia is multi-faceted, including therapy, nutrition education, and health monitoring. In extreme cases, self-starvation can lead to electrolyte imbalances, heart rhythm disturbances, and dehydration, which require hospitalization. During recovery, vital signs, electrolytes, and other physical conditions are monitored frequently, and ongoing therapy may be needed to prevent relapse.

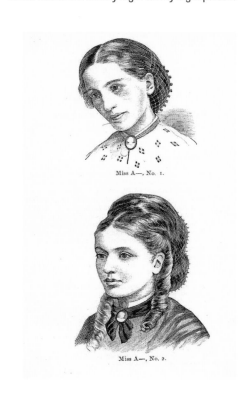

Two illustrations of photos taken in 1866 and 1870 showing the countenance of Miss A before and after anorexia treatment. She was a patient of William Withey Gull, who used these illustrations in his 1873 paper "Anorexia Nervosa" to first describe and categorize anorexia as a medical condition.

Using cannabis as a treatment for anorexia is a fairly new idea, although it has proven to be very effective for those whose anorexia is a result of cancer or HIV/AIDS. But there are reasons to believe the drug could be a promising treatment for the disorder, besides its penchant for causing "the munchies." A small Belgian study in 2011 found that those suffering from eating disorders have disfunction and imbalances with the body's endocannabinoid system, suggesting that

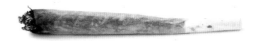

While it certainly seems as if medicinal marijuana can have a place in helping anorexics recover, the drug should be used in conjunction with other recovery methods, like cognitive behavioral therapy. With the right combination of treatments, cannabis may provide hope for a condition that often seems hopeless.

treatment with cannabinoids could help correct these defects. And a study in Denmark showed that anorexic patients receiving dronabinol—the synthetic form of THC—gained more weight than patients on a placebo.

Cannabis also increases sensitivity to smells and tastes, which can elevate the pleasure of eating, something anorexia sufferers often lose. And as anxiety is often a trigger for anorexic behavior, marijuana's antianxiety properties can be especially helpful. People who have used cannabis to overcome their anorexia report that using the drug helped them feel less self-conscious and less worried about counting calories.

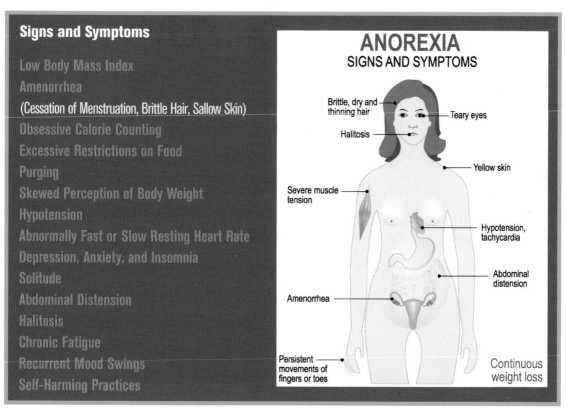

Signs and Symptoms

Low Body Mass Index
Amenorrhea
(Cessation of Menstruation, Brittle Hair, Sallow Skin)
Obsessive Calorie Counting
Excessive Restrictions on Food
Purging
Skewed Perception of Body Weight
Hypotension
Abnormally Fast or Slow Resting Heart Rate
Depression, Anxiety, and Insomnia
Solitude
Abdominal Distension
Halitosis
Chronic Fatigue
Recurrent Mood Swings
Self-Harming Practices

ANOREXIA
SIGNS AND SYMPTOMS

Brittle, dry and thinning hair
Teary eyes
Halitosis
Yellow skin
Severe muscle tension
Hypotension, tachycardia
Abdominal distension
Amenorrhea
Persistent movements of fingers or toes
Continuous weight loss

Depression, Anxiety, and Stress

We all feel sad or stressed out now and then; the struggles of life make sure of it! But for some individuals, those moods begin to feel overwhelming and last for weeks or months at a time, preventing them from living life to the fullest. Depression is characterized by several symptoms, including a depressive mood, lack of energy, feelings of worthlessness, lack of focus, and sleeping disorders. People who suffer with the condition can also be irritable, eat too much (or not enough), feel anxious, or even have physical symptoms like headaches, joint pain, or digestive trouble. And depression can make other physical issues—especially chronic pain—feel even worse.

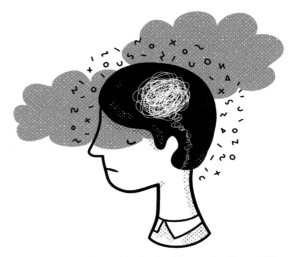

According to *The Oxford Handbook of Depression Comorbidity*, two to seven percent of people suffering from major depression die of suicide.

The disorder can affect anyone, although women are twice as likely as men to be depressed. And experts believe genetics play a role: If you have a parent who has struggled with depression, you are more likely to experience it. The cause of the disorder is still unknown, but doctors believe it may be connected to altered brain chemistry. Communication between brain cells that regulate mood may work less efficiently in those with depression, causing an imbalance of the neurotransmitters serotonin, norepinephrine, and dopamine.

Traditionally Treating Depression

With mild to moderate depression, talk therapy can often help, as it aims to change thoughts and behaviors that contribute to the feelings, or helps sufferers work through issues with relationships or unresolved issues. Exercise can also be a great way to help stave off mild depression, as it increases mood-boosting endorphins, plus helps increase energy and improve sleep. Other depression-busters include maintaining a supportive social circle (whether that be friends and family, support groups, or taking classes at a gym), or even adopting a pet—studies have shown that pet owners have better overall health than those who don't have a furry friend.

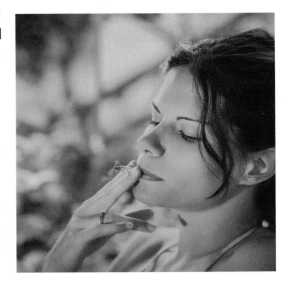

But for those who don't find relief through these channels, medications may be prescribed that help to balance the neurotransmitters in the brain. These antidepressants may take several weeks to take effect, and can come with many unpleasant side effects, such as nausea, weight gain, fatigue, irritability, or constipation. Worse yet, antidepressants may eventually stop working for some people, leading to more medications, and in younger people, antidepressants can actually increase suicidal thoughts and behavior.

Treating Depression With Marijuana

Studies of using cannabis for depression are relatively new, but there's plenty of anecdotal evidence to back up its effectiveness. Scientists are discovering that the drug works with the body's own endocannabinoid system to stabilize mood. And marijuana's effects on stress and anxiety are well-documented, with many studies showing that it decreases these feelings, which often go hand-in-hand with bouts of depression.

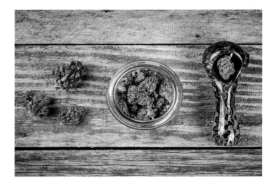

One thing to be aware of is that cannabis should only be used in small doses to fight depression; large doses have been known to have the opposite effect. For this reason, experts recommend "microdosing" when using cannabis to treat depression. Start with the smallest dose needed to have an effect—this is usually between three and ten mg of THC. And about a quarter of individuals can use even less than three mg. Because of these "microdoses," the best consumption method is edibles because they are easier to measure and control ingestion.

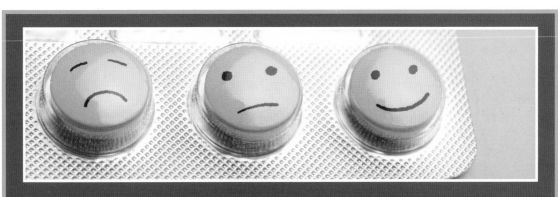

SSRIs

SSRIs (selective serotonin reuptake inhibitors) are the most widely prescribed antidepressants in most countries, although the actual biological mechanism by which they operate is unknown. SSRIs can be prescribed for anxiety, obsessive compulsive disorder, stroke recovery, and depression. Although they are found to be effective, they have a number of worrisome side effects, including suicidal thoughts and sexual dysfunction.

Nausea

We all felt it: that queasy, uneasy feeling in your stomach that makes the thought of food unbearable. If you're lucky, the feeling will eventually resolve on its own; but if you're unlucky, a bout of vomiting may soon follow. Like pain—which prevents us from doing things like touching hot stoves or working out too hard at the gym—nausea is our body's way of preventing more harm. If we eat a few bites of food and start feeling sick, that nausea prevents us from continuing to eat the food that is causing distress. Nausea and vomiting probably protected our early ancestors from eating poisonous plants or toxic foods.

The symptom is very non-specific, meaning it can be caused by a myriad of issues. Some common causes include motion sickness, food poisoning, pregnancy, and infections like the flu. Usually the condition is short-lived, resolving within a day or two. But in some cases, nausea can become chronic, causing a disruption to normal, everyday life. This can occur due to liver or kidney disease, irritable bowel syndrome, chemotherapy, brain tumors, inner ear conditions, or even stress and anxiety.

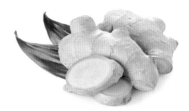

Ginger is a good natural remedy you can use to control nauseous sensations.

Causes of Nausea

Gastrointestinal Infections

Food Poisoning

Medications

(Chemotherapy, Antibiotics, Digoxin, Oral Contraceptives)

Pregnancy

Depression

Anxiety Disorders

Inner-Ear Diseases

(Motion sickness, Malignancy)

Inflammatory Diseases

(Celiac, Pancreatitis, Appendicitis)

Thyroid or Parathyroid Diseases

Uremia

Adrenal Insufficiency

Alcohol

Liver Failure

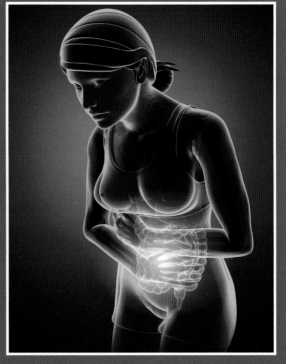

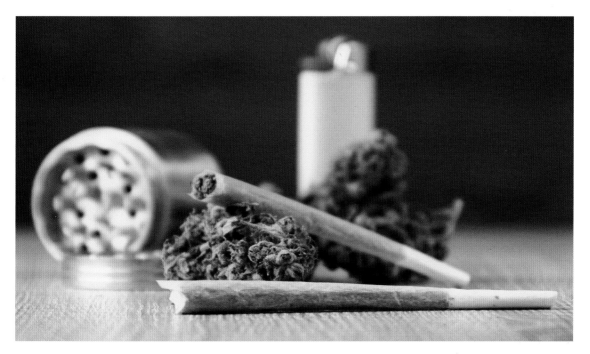

Inhalation methods are usually preferred by those suffering from nausea, since they are fast-acting, but tinctures are also a good option. Edibles can take much too long to take effect for someone desperate for relief from a queasy stomach, and attempting to swallow them can be impossible when the thought of food is unbearable. It should be noted, however, that heavy cannabis use—generally twenty times a month or more—can sometimes cause nausea. As with all drugs, moderation and responsible use is key.

Treating Nausea

When nausea is persistent, finding a way to get rid of it becomes a priority. Anti-nausea medications may be prescribed, but these can result in side effects that are just as unpleasant as the nausea itself. Diarrhea, constipation, headaches, and sleeping problems are all common. And many anti-nausea drugs are not meant to be taken for more than a few days, so if the underlying issue causing the nausea hasn't been resolved, the queasy feeling can come right back.

While cannabis has not been widely studied as a treatment for some conditions, nausea is one condition that has been repeatedly researched and treated with the drug. Its effectiveness at quelling the unpleasant feelings of the condition have been well-documented, with studies going back as far as the 1970s. *The New England Journal of Medicine* even published the results of a study more than forty years ago that described how cannabis was more successful at treating nausea and vomiting in chemotherapy patients than other drugs. And plenty of studies have followed, all coming to the same conclusion: Medicinal marijuana is an effective remedy to stop nausea in its tracks and increase appetite.

Post-Traumatic Stress Disorder

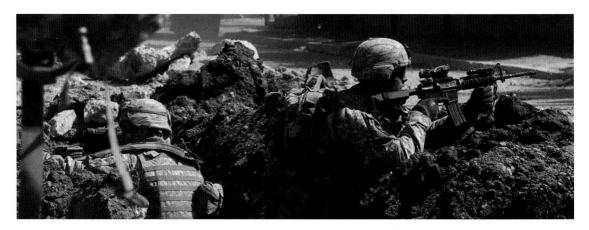

When we think of post-traumatic stress disorder, or PTSD, we often think of soldiers returning from war. And this is definitely a risk factor: Up to thirty percent of military personnel who have served in wars suffer from the disorder. But PTSD can affect anyone who has experienced frightening, life-threatening, or traumatic events, such as natural disasters, serious accidents, terrorist attacks, or sexual assault. It is estimated that about eight percent of Americans—around 24 million people—have PTSD at any given time.

Those who suffer from the disorder may have nightmares or flashbacks of their frightening experience, or may relive the trauma when confronted with reminders of the incident. This can cause them to avoid certain people, places, or activities that might trigger unwanted memories. Sufferers can develop depression, memory problems, personality changes, and issues with substance abuse—more than half of all men with PTSD have problems with alcohol. Eventually, these can impair the ability to function in normal social situations. Job loss, divorce, relationship issues and parenting problems are all common.

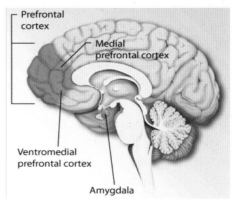

Post-Traumatic Stress Disorder is associated with several regions of the brain. Patients of PTSD often have less brain function in their ventromedial prefrontal cortex, which is responsible for experiencing and controlling emotions.

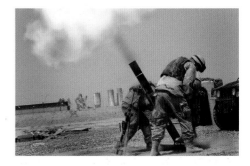

Traumatic events can cause our bodies to over-respond to traumatic events with too much adrenaline, creating deeply embedded neurological patterns that can make the person fearful of traumatic events in the future. Soldiers are constantly exposed to traumatic events of all sorts, including the detonation of artillery.

Treating PTSD

The main treatments for PTSD are therapy and medications like antidepressants or sleeping pills. Therapy aims to help people face and control their fears, as well as teaching relaxation and anger management skills. As a last resort, antipsychotic drugs may be prescribed, which can lead to weight gain, elevated cholesterol levels, muscle rigidity, and involuntary tremors—which may become permanent.

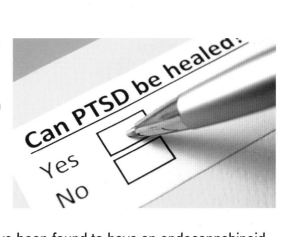

Interestingly, people suffering from PTSD have been found to have an endocannabinoid deficiency, making marijuana a great choice for treatment. Cannabis can fill in the gaps left by the missing endocannabinoids. And research has shown that the CBD in marijuana is especially effective at helping PTSD sufferers become desensitized to triggers that remind them of their past experience. CBD has also been shown to disrupt the recollection of long-term memories, helping them fade into the background.

Those who have used medicinal cannabis for PTSD say that unlike prescription medications, which "numb" feelings and make it impossible to process past trauma, cannabis allows them to feel their emotions in a way that is bearable, enabling them to process trauma safely.

Those who are unaccustomed to using marijuana may find that the THC in the drug aggravates the anxiety that comes along with PTSD; for this reason, it's recommended to look for a high-CBD strain if consuming it for the disorder. If an inhalation method is used, take just one hit and wait twenty minutes to see what kinds of effects it has. If using concentrates or edibles, start with a very small amount—then increase the dosage if necessary. Although cannabis alone cannot reverse the damage of PTSD—regular therapy should be a part of any treatment plan—it shows definite promise as a tool to provide relief for those who are suffering.

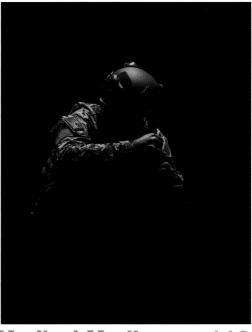

Insomnia

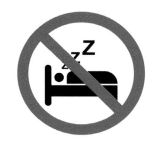

There are few things as frustrating as feeling tired and exhausted but being unable to sleep. You lie down in a nice, comfy bed at the end of the day, close your eyes, and … stay awake for hours. This maddening condition is insomnia, and it is defined as having difficulty falling asleep or staying asleep, even when you have ample opportunity to do so.

Acute insomnia affects all of us now and then. It can happen when we're worrying about an upcoming event, like a final exam or a big work presentation, or feeling distressed over bad news or events. Between thirty and forty percent of Americans report experiencing acute insomnia each year, but usually, this sort of sleep disruption resolves quickly, without the need for any treatment.

But chronic insomnia, which affects between ten and fifteen percent of Americans, occurs much more often—at least three nights per week, lasting at least three months. Causes can include a change in environment, work schedules, poor sleeping habits, or certain medications. Medical conditions like chronic pain, acid reflux, asthma, or Parkinson's disease can also affect sleep.

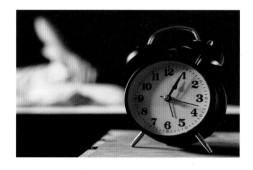

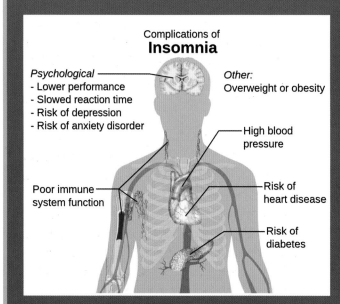

Complications of
Insomnia

Psychological
- Lower performance
- Slowed reaction time
- Risk of depression
- Risk of anxiety disorder

Other:
Overweight or obesity

High blood pressure

Poor immune system function

Risk of heart disease

Risk of diabetes

Complications of Insomnia

Those who suffer from insomnia often wake up earlier than they'd like and experience fatigue and sleepiness during the day. They may also feel irritable and anxious, have difficulty concentrating, and endure headaches and gastrointestinal issues. Even worse, a person with insomnia may be particularly uncoordinated and accident-prone in their sleep-deprived state, putting them at higher risk for injuries and making driving and certain other tasks more dangerous than usual.

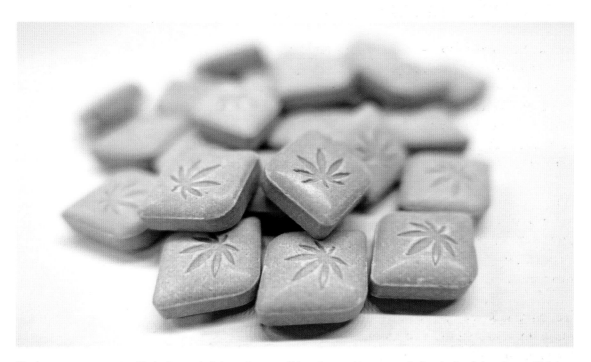

The best way to use cannabis for insomnia is ingesting an edible, taken an hour or two before bed so it has time to kick in. Since the effect of edibles lasts longer than other consumption methods, this can prevent restful sleep from being disrupted. It's also helpful to pair cannabis with relaxing aromatherapy scents, like lavender or chamomile.

Treating Insomnia

Many treatments for insomnia employ common sense to help induce sleep. These include exercising, maintaining a regular sleep schedule, avoiding caffeine close to bedtime, and making the sleeping area as comfortable as possible. It's also good to avoid watching television or eating in bed, ensuring that there are no unnecessary distractions. Some people also find it helpful to practice meditation or muscle relaxation techniques. When these measures fail, over-the-counter sleep aids, antihistamines (which often cause drowsiness), or prescription sleeping pills may be used.

But for those who have tried home remedies and still have trouble sleeping (but would rather not pop pills every night), cannabis may provide the ticket they need for a full night's sleep. Strains that have a low CBD content are best, as CBD has been found to have an energizing effect. THC, on the other hand, provides more of a feeling of relaxation. And it's interesting to note that older cannabis may work even better than fresh when using it for sleep: Over time, THC degrades into cannabinol (CBN), which has been shown to be five times more sedating than the original compound. This conversion doesn't happen quickly, however; it can literally take years for the CBN to form. So if you happen to have a stash of forgotten marijuana somewhere, it may make an excellent sedative!

Crohn's Disease

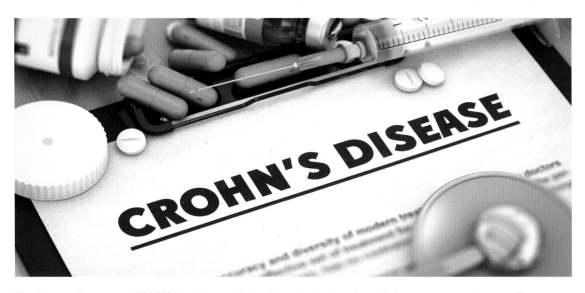

The disease affects around 780,000 Americans, with the diagnosis distributed equally between men and women. The causes of Crohn's are not well understood, but researchers believe a combination of genetics and environmental factors play a roll. Also, you are more likely to have the disease if a parent or sibling also has it.

Crohn's disease is a type of inflammatory bowel disease that can affect any part of the digestive tract, although it most commonly attacks the end of the small intestine and beginning of the large intestine. The disease can affect one area while leaving another alone, causing patches of diseased intestine between healthy parts.

In a normal gastrointestinal tract, friendly bacteria are present that help aid in digestion—the immune system knows not to attack these harmless bugs. But in the case of Crohn's disease, the bacteria are mistakenly seen as invaders, and the immune system responds, resulting in inflammation. Eventually, the inflammation becomes chronic, leading to thickened intestinal walls, ulcerations, and unpleasant symptoms. These can include persistent diarrhea, blood in the stools, abdominal cramps and pain, and an urgent need to use the bathroom. Loss of appetite, fatigue, and low energy are also common.

As a chronic disease, Crohn's can disrupt sufferers' lives in multiple ways. The need to always be near a bathroom can mean fewer social activities and result in isolation from friends or family. It is estimated that about half of sufferers miss an average of twenty-six days of work per year. This costs employers more than $1 billion in lost productivity, and those who suffer from the disease often worry about job security—many even hide their condition from their employer, fearing it will cost them their job or promotions. And the unpredictability of sudden flare-ups can cause constant stress—which, ironically, is thought to be a possible trigger for flare-ups!

Crohn's disease

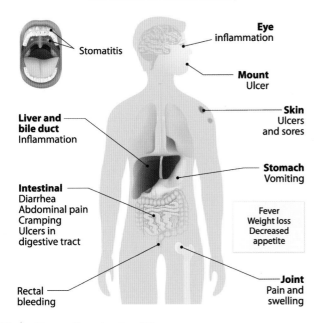

Eye inflammation

Stomatitis

Mount Ulcer

Liver and bile duct Inflammation

Skin Ulcers and sores

Stomach Vomiting

Intestinal
Diarrhea
Abdominal pain
Cramping
Ulcers in
digestive tract

Fever
Weight loss
Decreased
appetite

Rectal bleeding

Joint
Pain and
swelling

Crohn's can even cause "systemic" complications, which are issues outside of the digestive system. These include arthritis, skin problems, vitamin deficiencies, kidney stones, and liver disease. And the medications often given to Crohn's patients can result in serious side effects.

Treating Crohn's Disease

Treatment for this frustrating disease can often include many different medications, such as anti-inflammatory drugs, corticosteroids, immune system modifiers, antibiotics, and nutritional supplements. Surgery is an unfortunate necessity for up to seventy-five percent of Crohn's patients, and can consist of removing the diseased parts of intestine and joining healthy ends together. While this surgery can help people remain symptom-free for years, it does not cure the disease, and Crohn's may eventually rear its ugly head once more.

While Crohn's has no cure, more and more studies are beginning to show that cannabis can be an effective way to alleviate some of the symptoms of this disruptive disease. We already know some of medicinal marijuana's amazing properties: it is anti-inflammatory, reduces pain, lowers anxiety, calms nausea, and increases appetite. All of which can be huge benefits for Crohn's sufferers. The cannabinoids in marijuana help the immune system stop its attack against healthy tissue, while at the same time providing pain relief and helping increase appetite.

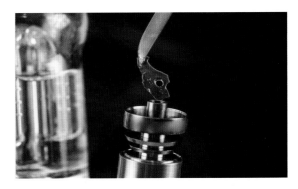

The anecdotal evidence emerging from those who have tried cannabis for the disease has been extremely encouraging, with some saying the drug even helped them reach remission. Concentrated oil has been a favorite method of consumption for Crohn's sufferers who choose to use cannabis.

Multiple Sclerosis

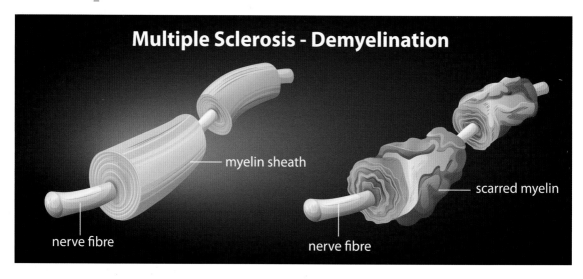

Multiple Sclerosis - Demyelination

myelin sheath

scarred myelin

nerve fibre

nerve fibre

A combination of environmental and genetic conditions can contribute to the development of MS, although the actual cause is not known. Strangely, the rate of MS is more common among people who live farther away from the equator than people who live closer to the equator. Also, there is some debate as to whether microbes and infectious agents have a cause in the development of MS.

A nother example of the immune system going haywire is multiple sclerosis. "Sclerosis" refers to a hardening of tissue—in this case, the fatty substance that surrounds and protects nerve fibers, called myelin. In this disease, the immune system causes inflammation that damages or destroys myelin, leaving behind scar tissue in multiple areas. When this happens, messages within the central nervous system are altered or even stopped, resulting in a variety of neurological symptoms.

The process of constructing myelin in the body is called myelination. Myelination begins sheathing the nerves of a person while they are still in utero during the third trimester. The process begins to accelerate in the first year of life, correlating with the child's fast development.

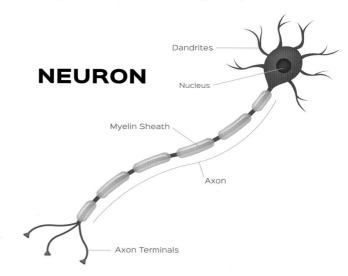

NEURON

Dandrites

Nucleus

Myelin Sheath

Axon

Axon Terminals

Symptoms of MS

Symptoms of the disease vary from person to person and can be random and unpredictable, making it difficult at times to definitively diagnose the disorder. But some of the most common symptoms include fatigue, weakness, numbness or tingling in the face, body, or extremities, walking difficulties, muscle spasms, dizziness, and vision problems. Depression is also an extremely common symptom—in fact, depression is more common in MS patients than in the general population or among those with other chronic conditions.

Less common symptoms can include speech problems, tremors, difficulty swallowing, breathing problems, and seizures. Secondary symptoms can also arise as a result of the primary symptoms of the disease; for instance, a difficulty with walking can result in weakened muscles or a loss of bone density. MS sufferers may also eventually be unable to continue working, or feel that dealing with their disease leaves them isolated from family and friends.

There is an absolutely astonishing amount of symptoms that are associated with recognizing and diagnosing multiple sclerosis. Any number of neurological signs occur during the disease's onset, including automatic, visual, motor, and sensory problems topping the list. Sufferers of MS may feel a lack or change in sensory perception, tingling, numbness, muscle spasms, weakness, and blurred vision.

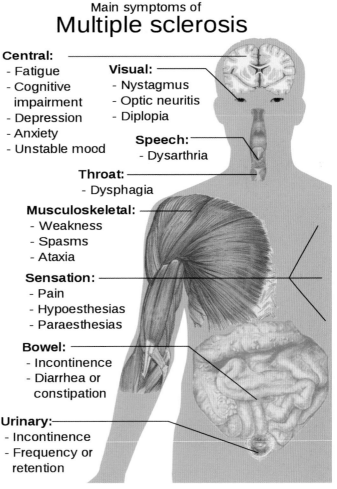

Main symptoms of
Multiple sclerosis

Central:
- Fatigue
- Cognitive impairment
- Depression
- Anxiety
- Unstable mood

Visual:
- Nystagmus
- Optic neuritis
- Diplopia

Speech:
- Dysarthria

Throat:
- Dysphagia

Musculoskeletal:
- Weakness
- Spasms
- Ataxia

Sensation:
- Pain
- Hypoesthesias
- Paraesthesias

Bowel:
- Incontinence
- Diarrhea or constipation

Urinary:
- Incontinence
- Frequency or retention

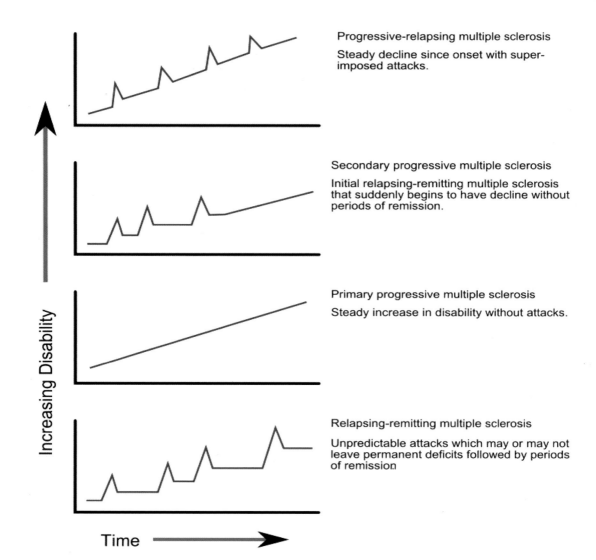

Increasing Disability

Progressive-relapsing multiple sclerosis
Steady decline since onset with superimposed attacks.

Secondary progressive multiple sclerosis
Initial relapsing-remitting multiple sclerosis that suddenly begins to have decline without periods of remission.

Primary progressive multiple sclerosis
Steady increase in disability without attacks.

Relapsing-remitting multiple sclerosis
Unpredictable attacks which may or may not leave permanent deficits followed by periods of remission

Time

Types of multiple sclerosis and how they progress.

Diagnosing and Treating MS

The disease generally begins with a single first episode, known as Clinically Isolated Syndrome (CIS). CIS is characteristic of MS, but does not always develop into the disease. If another episode occurs, an official diagnosis of MS may be made. Most patients—about eighty-five percent—are afflicted with Relapse-Remitting MS (RRMS), which consists of periods of symptom-free remissions interspersed with episodes of new or worsening symptoms. But eventually, the disease can progress to the point of fewer remissions and a steady deterioration of symptoms.

MS has no cure, so treatments aim to control symptoms. The most commonly prescribed drugs are corticosteroids, which reduce inflammation and suppress the immune system to prevent it from attacking healthy tissue. A number of drugs can also be prescribed to slow the progression of the disease, and these can either be injected, taken in pill form, or administered by intravenous infusion. Physical therapy is often used to help patients restore coordination and strengthen muscles.

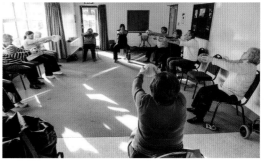

Physical therapy is often used to help patients restore coordination and strengthen muscles.

Marijuana and MS

Fortunately, there's one more option MS patients can turn to—medicinal cannabis. About a quarter of all MS patients have tried the drug to control their symptoms, and even the American Academy of Neurology has concluded that cannabis can be a helpful tool for controlling pain and muscle spasms. Lending a bit of celebrity to the fight against MS, former talk show host Montel Williams, who was diagnosed in 1999, has been using medicinal cannabis to control his disease for more than seventeen years, and has become a vocal proponent for using the plant as medicine. Not only does cannabis help decrease pain and muscle spasms, but it can relieve the depression that so often plagues MS sufferers. Williams even attempted to kill himself by jumping in front of a New York City taxi after he was first diagnosed, and now credits the drug for changing his life.

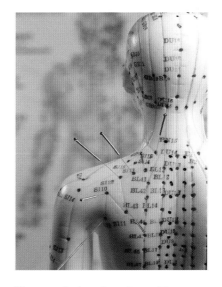

Many people throughout the world use alternative methods to treat MS, although many of these methods have no or little proven effect. These methods include vitamin D treatment, yoga, acupuncture, relaxation, meditation, hyperbaric oxygen therapy, and herbal medicine.

Two synthetic forms of marijuana are FDA-approved for MS patients, and can be taken in capsule form by mouth. But experts think the "real deal" could be even more effective for treating symptoms. They recommend using a high-CBD strain of cannabis to help with the pain, fatigue, and depression, with edibles and topicals being popular choices. Or, go with Williams' favorite consumption method, vaporizing. Williams also wants to share the plant's power with others: He is so confident that medicinal cannabis is a drug of the future that he's launched his own line of cannabis products that are available online and at more than thirty dispensaries in California.

ADHD

We all know a kid or two who can be a bit rambunctious now and then—it's what kids do. But for up to eleven percent of children—and five percent of adults—behavior and feelings can reach a point where they disrupt normal life and make it difficult to function at school, home, work, or with friends.

Diagnosing Attention Deficit Hyperactivity Disorder

There are three types of ADHD: an inattentive type, a hyperactivity/impulsive type, and a combination type. As the name suggests, the inattentive type is characterized by an inability to pay attention. Those who have this type of ADHD may have a hard time staying focused on tasks, make careless mistakes, fail to follow instructions, and can be disorganized, distracted, and forgetful. With the hyperactivity/impulsive type of ADHD, it's not uncommon to see fidgety behavior, an inability to sit still, running or climbing when it's not appropriate, and talking at inopportune times.

Diagnosing ADHD in children requires an evaluation with a pediatrician or psychiatrist with experience in the disorder. They will gather information about behavior from parents and teachers, and perform a medical evaluation to rule out any medical problems like hearing or vision disorders. Adults are often unaware that they have the disorder, and may have a history of job troubles or difficult relationships. Adults can use ADHD symptom checklists to see if they may have the condition, and talk to their doctor about a diagnosis.

Approximate Prevalence Distribution of the Subtypes of ADHD

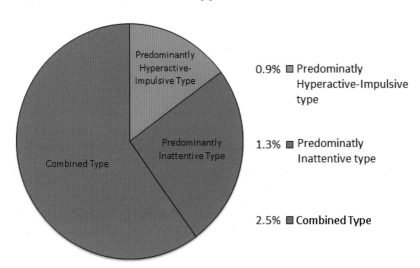

0.9% ☐ Predominatly Hyperactive-Impulsive type

1.3% ☐ Predominatly Inattentive type

2.5% ☐ Combined Type

Of the total population of adults that suffer from ADHD (almost five percent of the population), nineteen percent suffer from hyperactive symptoms.

Sign of Inattentive ADHD

Forgetful and Distracted

Not Responsive

Cannot Sustain Attention

No Attention to Detail

Difficulty Organizing Information

Avoids Tasks That Require Concentration (adult)

Procrastinates (adult)

Difficulty Multitasking (adult)

Poor Time Management (adult)

Indecisive and Hesitant to Execute (adult)

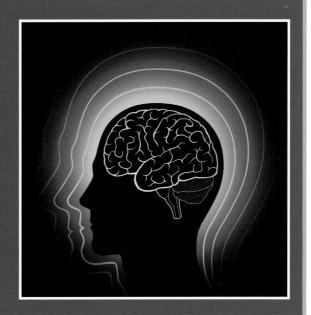

Signs of Hyperactive/Impulsive ADHD

Squirms and Fidgets

Excessive Talking

Excessive Need to Be Active

Interrupts Conversations and Intrudes

Avoids Sedentary Work (adult)

Needs Constant Activity (adult)

Easily Bored (adult)

Impatient (adult)

Easily Irritated (adult)

Impulsive and Irresponsible (adult)

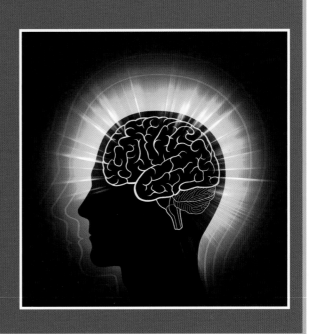

Treating ADHD

Treatment for ADHD is usually a combination of education, psychotherapy, and medication. Surprisingly, the most common medications for the disorder are stimulants. It may seem counterproductive to use a stimulant to help someone focus or to calm fidgety behavior, but the brains of those with ADHD tend to be deficient in the neurotransmitters dopamine and norepinephrine; the stimulants increase these neurotransmitters. But the medications used to treat ADHD—like Ritalin and Adderall—have been known to cause many side effects, such as nervousness, insomnia, high blood pressure, or a decrease in appetite.

And there's another problem with so many kids and young adults using these drugs: Between three and eight percent of high school seniors have admitted to using the drugs without a prescription, using them as a way to improve mental focus before big exams. Some teenagers have even faked ADHD symptoms in order to get the drugs!

Cannabis has the same effect on dopamine levels as stimulants, so it would stand to reason that it could work to combat the symptoms of ADHD. Still, research into the effectiveness of the drug for the disorder is in its very early stages. But many who suffer from ADHD swear by marijuana's ability to help them focus. For children, CBD oil is recommended as the oil once or twice a day can help their kids feel calmer and less irritable. This, in conjunction with behavioral therapy or stress management techniques, can lead to a much more productive life with ADHD.

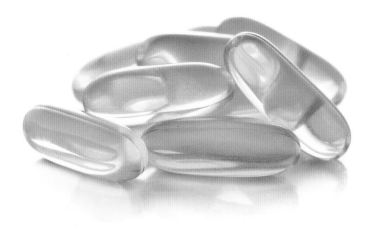

A 2013 study published by *The Journal of Psychiatry* found that one third of their testing group of children with ADHD had improved after their diets were modified with fatty acid supplementation and artificial food coloring restriction. Although, the study also found that the children who benefited most from these modifications were children who already had restricted diets due to sensitivities.

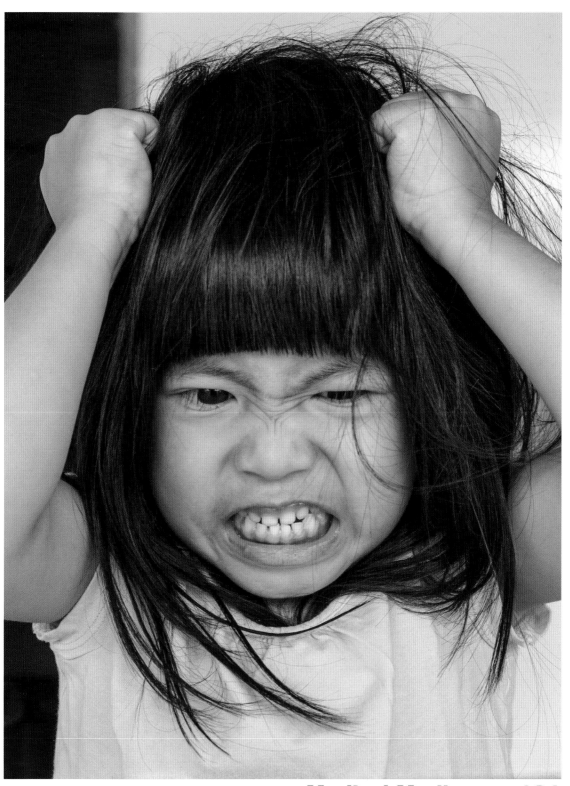

Epilepsy

The fourth most common neurological disorder, epilepsy is characterized by unpredictable and recurrent seizures due to a surge of electrical activity in the brain. This surge of activity causes a disruption in the messages sent by the brain to other areas of the body. The disorder affects 3.4 million Americans, including around 470,000 children, and for about one third of those people, available treatments are ineffective. The cause of epilepsy is often completely unknown, although occasionally it can be a result of brain trauma or a family history of the disease.

Epilepsy can be caused by serious brain trauma, like strokes or tumors, or from previous infections. There are some genetic factors can cause epilepsy, but more than fifty percent of epilepsy cases are caused by unknown factors, according to the National Institute for Health and Clinical Excellence.

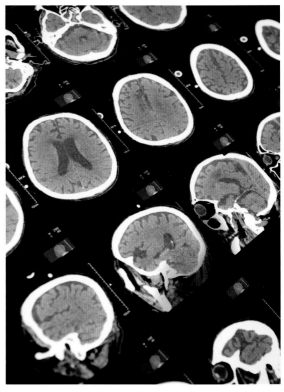

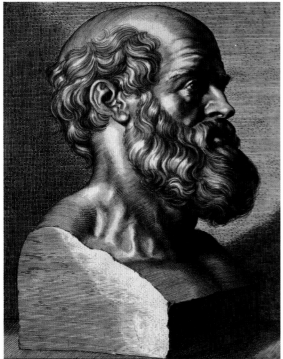

Hippocrates of Kos, the Greek physician who is a seminal figure in the history of medicine, was one of the first notable people to reject the popular antiquarian view that epilepsy was a sacred disease caused by the gods. The ancient Greeks thought of epilepsy as a type of spiritual possession that they associated with both genius and divine intervention. It was often associated with the moon goddess, Selene, who would afflict people with the sacred disease if she was not happy with them. Hippocrates later disputed such assumptions in his work *On the Sacred Disease*, where he claimed that epilepsy was not divine in origin, but stemmed from a treatable disease of the brain.

Categorizing Epilepsy

Seizures are categorized in three different groups. "Generalized onset" seizures affect both sides of the brain at the same time. "Focal onset" seizures affect one area on one side of the brain; a person experiencing a focal onset seizure may either be awake and aware, or confused or unaware of what is happening. "Unknown onset" seizures are of unknown origin—seizures that occur at night or to someone who lives alone may at first be categorized this way; but after more information is learned, they may be placed into the "generalized" or "focal" categories.

Some of the symptoms of generalized and focal onset seizures are similar—both can result in motor symptoms like jerking movements, muscles becoming either weak and limp or rigid and tense, and muscle twitching and spasms. Generalized onset seizures can also have non-motor symptoms called absence seizures. Absence seizures do not cause the dramatic muscle twitches often associated with epilepsy, but rather are categorized by lapses in awareness and staring. They are more common in children than adults, and can be so brief that they are sometimes mistaken for daydreaming. Focal onset seizures can have non-motor symptoms as well, which manifest as changes in sensation, emotions, thinking, or autonomic functions such as waves of heat or cold, goosebumps, or a racing heart.

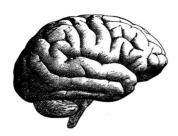

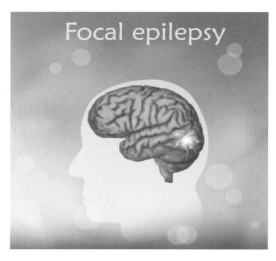

There are two types of focal onset seizures: focal onset aware and focal onset impaired awareness. Focal aware seizures often affect the temporal lobes and precede more traumatic generalized seizures. Those who suffer from focal awareness seizures stay conscious. Focal impaired seizures often affect larger sections of the hemisphere and cause the sufferer to lose consciousness.

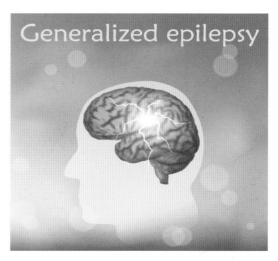

Generalized seizures affect both hemispheres of the brain and impair consciousness. There are many types of seizures that are categorized under the generalized seizure umbrella, including absence seizures, myoclonic seizures, clonic seizures, tonic-clonic seizures, and atonic seizures.

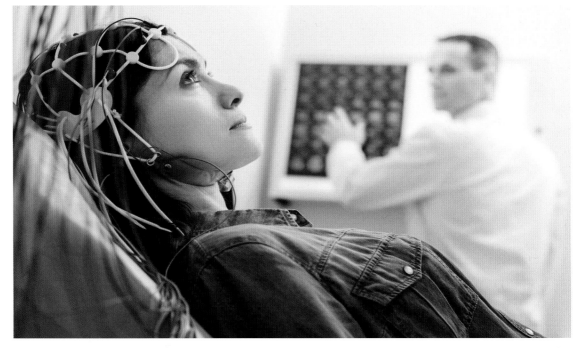

An electroencephalogram (EEG) is a test that can monitor the activity of your brains waves and can help in the diagnosis of epilepsy and epileptic seizures. They can also be used to determine whether the seizure a patient is experiencing is a focal onset or generalized onset seizure.

Treating Epilepsy

Epilepsy can be a very disruptive disorder, causing issues with school or work, and affecting a person's ability to drive or live alone. Those with epilepsy are more susceptible to depression and anxiety, can have learning disabilities, may have problems sleeping, and are at risk for falls and injuries. There is no cure for the disorder, but sufferers have several treatment options. Anti-epileptic drugs are usually the first course of action, but if those don't work, surgery may be a possibility. Surgery is especially helpful for those whose seizures are a result of benign brain tumors or structural defects. Another option is an implantable neuromodulation device. These devices use small electrical currents to signal the malfunctioning nerve cells to work correctly.

Anti-epileptic drugs come with a laundry list of possible side effects, including dizziness, sleep issues, slurred speech, double vision, weight gain, loss of bone density, rashes, and memory problems. Some people find they simply can't tolerate the side effects of the drugs. And what about those one third of epilepsy sufferers who can't even find a treatment that works? For some of these people, cannabis has been the answer.

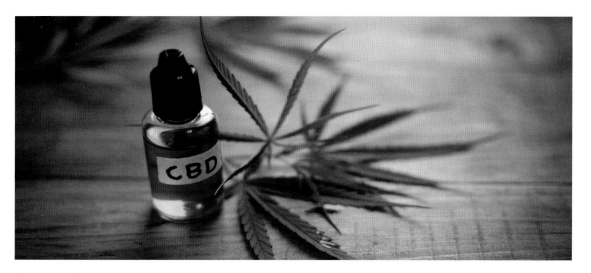

Cannabidiol (CBD) has shown to be very effective in preventing seizures in children, and was approved by the FDA in 2018 for treating Lennox–Gastaut syndrome, a childhood onset form of epilepsy, and Dravet sundrome, a form of epilepsy in which seizures are caused by hot temperatures or fevers.

Managing With Marijuana

Research has shown great promise for using medicinal cannabis for epilepsy, even for children. In fact, a high-CBD, low-THC strain of marijuana known as Charlotte's Web was named after a five-year-old girl named Charlotte Figi, whose severe epilepsy was brought under control using the strain in a concentrated oil.

A high CBD strain seems to be key in treating the disorder, as the cannabinoid affects the body in such a way that it reduces seizures. Plus, a low-THC strain ensures that those with epilepsy can control their seizures while still remaining clear-headed throughout their day. Oils and tinctures are popular consumption methods, although for adults, smoking or vaporization may be used for more immediate relief. But the advantage for using an oil or tincture is that a very precise dosage can be used—once the effective dose is found, it is easy to continue dosing the correct amount.

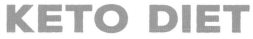

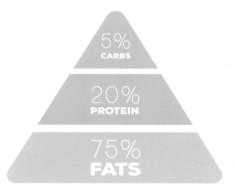

Aside from anticonvulsant medications and surgery for treating epilepsy, there have been some studies to show the effectiveness of a ketogenic diet for reducing the amount of seizures one experiences.

PMS

If you're a woman who experiences a few unpleasant or slightly bothersome symptoms in the days leading up to your period, you're definitely not alone. In fact, about ninety percent of women have at least a few premenstrual symptoms every month, but most of these are easily managed. However, for some women, the symptoms they endure can have an impact on their daily lives; when this happens, the symptoms are referred to as premenstrual syndrome, or PMS.

Symptoms of PMS

PMS is caused by hormone fluctuations that occur after ovulation. Estrogen and progesterone levels fall sharply until menstruation begins, at which point hormones start to rise again. This roller coaster of hormones can cause both physical and emotional symptoms. Cramps, headaches, breast tenderness, bloating, and constipation or diarrhea are all common physical symptoms associated with PMS. Emotionally, PMS can cause irritability, mood swings, crying spells, anxiety, and difficulty concentrating. Sleep problems and food cravings aren't uncommon, either.

E₁ Estrone

E₂ Estradiol

E₃ Estriol

E₄ Estetrol

Estrogen is a female sex hormone. There are four major types of estrogens, including estrone, estiril, estetrol, and estradiol.

Progesterone

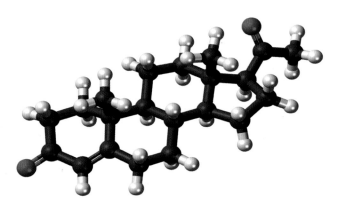

Progesterone is an endogenous steroid that plays a part in the menstrual cycle, pregnancy, and formation of the human embryo.

About five percent of women suffer from a more severe form of PMS known as premenstrual dysphoric disorder, or PMDD. The symptoms are much the same as in PMS, but are more serious and distressing. For instance, while irritability can be a symptom of both PMS and PMDD, in PMDD it can often lead to lasting anger and outbursts that affect other people. Women with PMDD are also prone to severe depression or even thoughts of suicide.

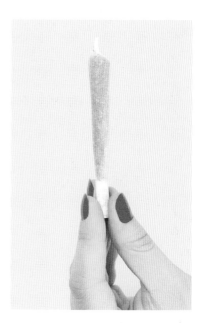

PMS can affect other conditions as well, like asthma, allergies, or migraines, which can all worsen in the days leading up to menstruation. And women with depression or anxiety disorders, chronic fatigue syndrome, or irritable bowel syndrome may also notice a worsening of symptoms during this time.

Diagnosing PMDD

The Diagnostic and Statistical Manual of Mental Disorders (5th Ed.) identifies seven criteria, each with various symptoms, that can be used to help diagnose PMDD. These criteria are labeled A through G and cover a variety of symptoms that can help identify the disorder. Some of these symptoms include:

Mood Swings
Irritability ˙
Depressed Mood
Lack of Interest in Usual Activities
Lacking the Ability to Concentrate
Lack of Energy
Food Cravings
Excessive Hunger
Hypersomnia or Insomnia
Increased Interpersonal Conflicts
Anxiety or Tension

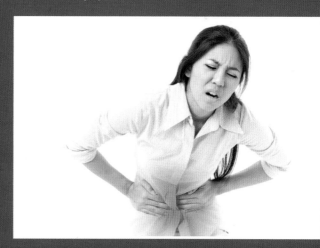

There are many other symptoms, and some of the criteria also state that these symptoms would also interfere with one's personal/work life, would not be considered an exacerbation of already diagnosed conditions like personality, depressive, or panic disorders, and are not tied to substance abuse or medication.

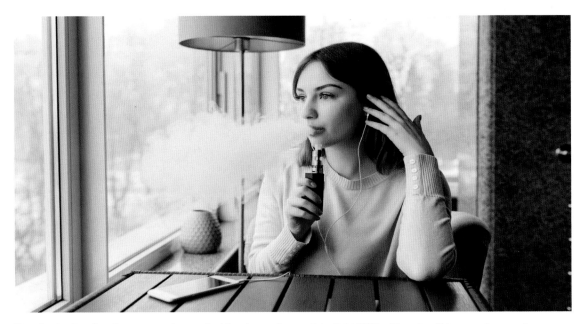

Vaporization is a favorite consumption method for those who use it to fight PMS, although edibles are also popular—especially cannabis-infused chocolate products. These are perfect if you're craving sweets but also need to stave off uncomfortable symptoms (just remember to wait and see how the product affects you before eating too much). For those who aren't squeamish, cannabis suppositories can be a great choice for relieving cramps and pain. There are even bath soaks and salts, infused with cannabis and essential oils, so you can immerse yourself in the comforting, pain-relieving properties of the plant.

Managing PMS

Fortunately, for many women, taking a few simple steps can go a long way in easing PMS symptoms. Getting regular exercise, clocking in eight hours of sleep a night, and not smoking are not only great ways to stay healthy in general, but they help to keep PMS symptoms at bay, as well. Avoiding caffeine, sugar, and salt in the two weeks between ovulation and menstruation can also help, as well as making use of meditation or yoga.

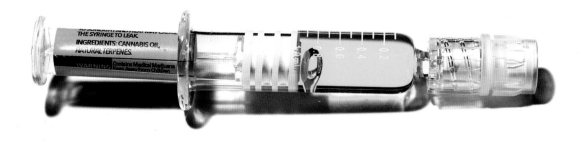

But if these don't do enough, certain medications may be taken, such as over-the-counter pain relievers, antidepressants, or antianxiety medication. Birth control pills can also sometimes provide relief, as they help to keep hormones on an even keel. Calcium and B and D vitamins have also been shown to ease some PMS symptoms, so taking supplements or eating foods containing these nutrients may help.

But when these avenues don't work—or for women who'd like to add an extra weapon to their arsenal—there's cannabis. Even England's Queen Victoria was known to use cannabis to relieve menstrual cramps —if it's good enough for a queen, it good enough for the rest of us! Obviously, medicinal marijuana's ability to calm cramps has already been documented; but the drug can also decrease breast tenderness, ease headaches, calm gastrointestinal issues, help promote sleep, and even stabilize mood.

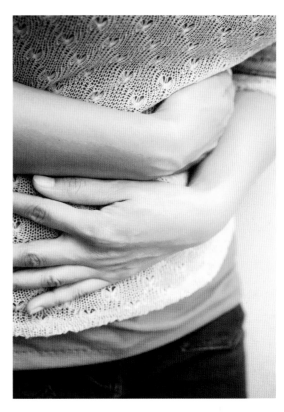

According to *American Family Physician*, only a small percentage of women who experience PMS have severe symptoms that cannot be managed easily.

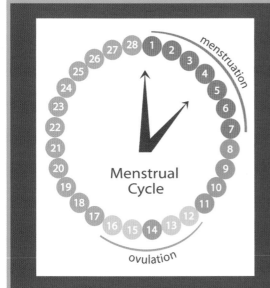

Other Ways to Manage

The *American Family Physician* cites some preliminary evidence that vitamin B6 and chasteberry can help with the management of menstrual pain, although it denies the effectiveness of other common herbal and natural remedies such as St. John's wort, soy, vitamin E, and saffron. *The Office of Women's Health* has also stated that anti-inflammatories like naproxen can help with the physical pain.

Alzheimer's Disease

The term Alzheimer's disease often makes us think of the elderly, but this progressive disease is not a normal part of aging. In fact, this irreversible brain disorder—which destroys memory, cognition, and even the ability to perform simple everyday tasks—does not even exclusively affect older people: About 200,000 Americans under the age of sixty-five are afflicted with Alzheimer's—the youngest person to ever be diagnosed was only twenty-seven years old.

The Symptoms of Alzheimer's Disease

The classic first symptoms are memory lapses, such as misplacing objects, struggling to remember the correct word, or forgetting names; the most common symptom is failing to retain newly learned information, because the disease first attacks the part of the brain responsible for learning. Unfortunately, Alzheimer's doesn't stop there. The disease marches through the brain, leading to increasingly severe symptoms, including disorientation, mood changes, serious memory loss, confusion about time or place, and an inability to recognize friends, family, or caregivers. Eventually, Alzheimer's patients reach a point where they are unable to care for themselves. They can have difficulty communicating, and may lose the ability to walk, sit up, or swallow, making them especially susceptible to infections like pneumonia.

While the biggest risk factors for Alzheimer's—age and a family history of the disease—can't be changed, researchers are discovering that there may be ways to prevent it. Living a healthy lifestyle is key—eating well, exercising, and avoiding tobacco and alcohol are a good start. There have also been studies linking heart health to brain health, so staying on top of heart issues like high blood pressure and high cholesterol is vital.

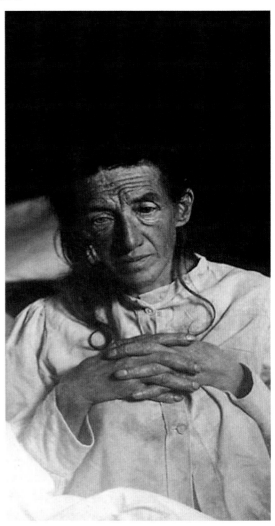

A picture of Auguste Deter in 1902, the first patient to ever be diagnosed with Alzheimer's disease.

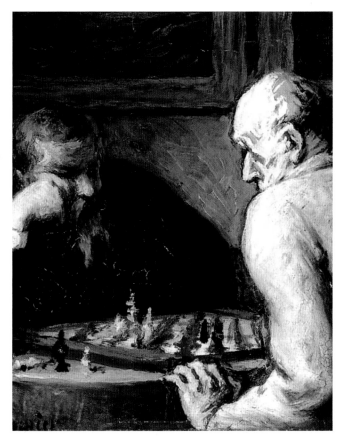

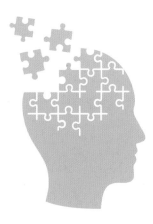

Activities such as playing chess or regular social interaction have been linked to a reduced risk of developing Alzheimer's disease.

Diagnosing Alzheimer's can be very difficult, but it is often successfully diagnosed after the cognitive impairments of the disease begin to compromise the daily routine of those who suffer from it. Alzheimer's significantly affects the lives of those who suffer from it, and the lifespans of those who are diagnosed are greatly reduced. After diagnosis, the lifespan of those who are suffering from the disease is three to ten years. Less than three percent of people living with Alzheimer's live longer than fourteen years after diagnosis.

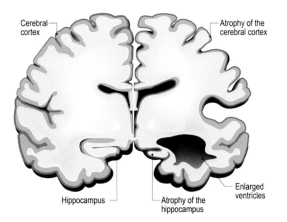

Healthy

Alzheimer's disease

Cerebral cortex

Atrophy of the cerebral cortex

Hippocampus

Atrophy of the hippocampus

Enlarged ventricles

Alzheimer's atrophies various regions of the brain. The loss of neurons and synapses in the cerebral cortex and other subcortical regions are the prime causes of the degradation of the temporal and parietal lobe.

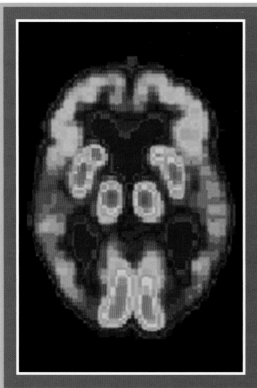

Preventing Alzheimer's Disease

There are a number of medical and recreational options one can partake in to help prevent Alzheimer's disease. Although there is no definitive evidence to support these claims, there are some results that are promising in tackling the problem of Alzheimer's. Lowering your exposure to cardiovascular risk factors like high cholesterol, smoking, diabetes, and hypertension could help lower your risk of developing Alzheimer's disease. Lifestyle changes can also have a tremendous effect in preventing the onset of Alzheimer's. Mentally and physically challenging activities like reading, puzzles, games, playing musical instruments, socializing, and exercising have all been show to lower the likelihood of developing Alzheimer's and reducing the severity of the disease's symptoms. Healthy diets, including Japanese and Mediterranean diets, can also reduce your risk to developing the disease.

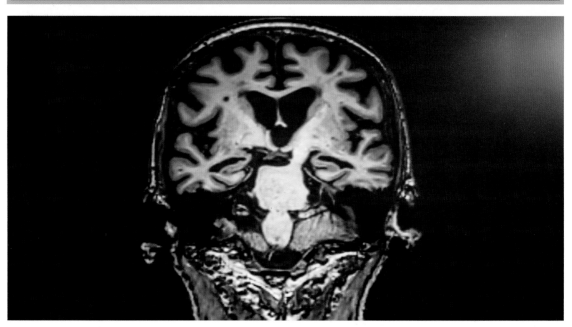

Alzheimer's is the most common cause of dementia—between sixty and eighty percent of all dementia cases can be attributed to the disease.

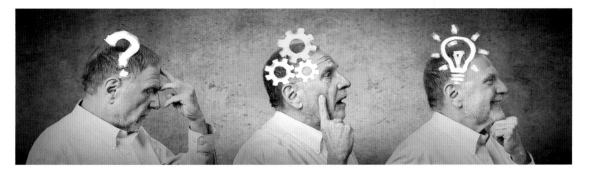

Since the majority of Alzheimer's patients are elderly, smoking cannabis isn't always the best consumption method—especially if the patient also has a lung disease like emphysema or chronic obstructive pulmonary disease. Oils or tinctures are a much easier route to take, although edibles can be a good choice, as well. As always, be careful with the dosing, and make sure to wait until the drug takes effect before deciding on a larger dose.

Treating Alzheimer's

So far, Alzheimer's has no cure, and there is no way to stop the eventual progression of the disease. But treatments are available to slow it down and to treat symptoms. Medications may be prescribed which prevent the breakdown of chemicals in the brain responsible for learning and memory. These can delay the loss of independence suffered by those with Alzheimer's, prolonging their quality of life. Other medications may also be given to relieve some of the symptoms that come along with the disease: Antidepressants can lift mood and decrease irritability, antianxiety medications can ease anxiety and restlessness, and antipsychotic medications can help with aggression, hostility, or hallucinations. Some patients also add supplements like coenzyme Q10, ginkgo biloba, coral calcium, or coconut oil to their diets, although research of these is limited and there is little evidence to support their effects on Alzheimer's.

There has, however, been some research into the effects of cannabis on Alzheimer's disease, and the findings are promising. The THC in marijuana has been shown to inhibit the buildup of proteins, called amyloid plaques, in the brains of Alzheimer's patients. When levels of these proteins are abnormally high, as they are in Alzheimer's patients, they can clump together and collect between neurons, disrupting cell function. Cannabis can also decrease the inflammation that occurs around these amyloid plaques. The other cannabinoids in marijuana show promising effects on the brain, as well. They may help prevent cell death, and may even stimulate cell growth in the area of the brain responsible for memory.

And of course, cannabis has already been shown to provide relief for some of the secondary symptoms that come along with Alzheimer's disease, like depression, anxiety, sleep disruptions, appetite changes, and irritability.

Parkinson's Disease

Parkinson's disease—another incurable and progressive brain disorder—affects about one million people in the United States. People with this disease tend to experience a wide range of differing symptoms; no two people with Parkinson's are alike. But all of those who suffer from this disease have one thing in common: A loss of dopamine-producing neurons in an area of the brain that is responsible for body movement and coordination. And it is not until a substantial number of these neurons die—about eighty percent—that symptoms begin to appear.

Symptoms of Parkinson's

Symptoms of Parkinson's usually begin slowly—early signs of the disease can be so mild that they go unnoticed. Sometimes the only indication that something is amiss is a slight tremor in one hand or a feeling of stiffness. Other symptoms include slowed movement, rigid muscles, impaired balance, or speech or writing changes. Some people also notice difficulty performing unconscious movements like swinging their arms when they walk.

Often the preliminary symptoms will begin on only one side of the body, but as the disease progresses, both sides of the body can be affected. Tremors and coordination become increasingly worse, and activities like walking, eating, and dressing can be difficult. Eventually, a walker or wheelchair may be needed, and those in the late stages of the disease often need round-the-clock care to function.

Most of those with Parkinson's disease first show symptoms after the age of fifty; but between two and ten percent of those with the disease are under the age of fifty. One of these patients, the actor Michael J. Fox—who was only twenty-nine years old when he was diagnosed—is now a proponent of medicinal cannabis for Parkinson's. His foundation—the Michael J. Fox Foundation—has been fighting for legal medicinal cannabis not only for Parkinson's, but for other disorders like multiple sclerosis and epilepsy, as well.

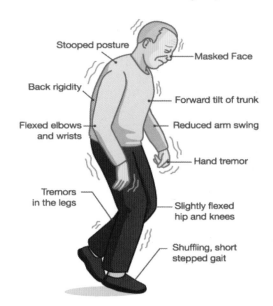

Parkinson's Disease Symptoms

Stooped posture

Masked Face

Back rigidity

Forward tilt of trunk

Flexed elbows and wrists

Reduced arm swing

Hand tremor

Tremors in the legs

Slightly flexed hip and knees

Shuffling, short stepped gait

PARKINSON'S DISEASE

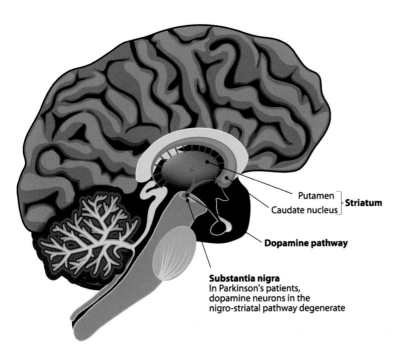

Putamen ⎤
Caudate nucleus ⎦ **Striatum**

Dopamine pathway

Substantia nigra
In Parkinson's patients, dopamine neurons in the nigro-striatal pathway degenerate

The degradation of motor and coordination skills is caused by the dieback of cells in the midbrain's substantia nigra, which is responsible for many functions like reward-seeking, learning, addiction, eye movement, and motor planning. The substantia nigra is mediated by the striatum, which relies on the substantia nigra's dopamine-related functions to operate. The striatum coordinates many functions related to the functions of the substantia nigra, including planning, decision making, motivation, reward cognition, and reinforcement.

Managing Parkinson's

Aside from turning toward surgery or medications to treat Parkinson's, there are more traditional options patients can use in order to maintain mobility and manage pain. According to the magazine *Parkinson's Disease*, there is scarce evidence that rehabilitation practices can improve mobility and speech difficulties. But patients under the care of a physiotherapist tend to manage better, and even exercise not supervised under the umbrella of physical rehabilitation can help patients remain mobile, flexible, and strong. The Lee Silverman voice treatment (LSVT) approach to treating speech impairments is widely practiced to help patients with their declining speech functions. Palliative care techniques can also be extremely useful in the early stages of the disease in order to help patients cope and transition healthily without too much of a decline in their quality of life after diagnosis.

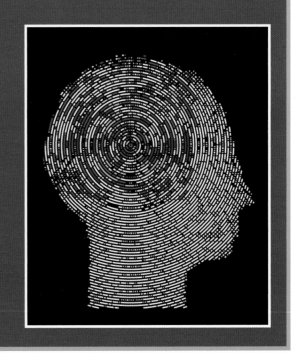

Treating Parkinson's

Treatments include prescription medications to replenish dopamine, which may temporarily reduce tremors and improve coordination, or other drugs that help to suppress the effects of the disease. If medications don't work, surgery may be an option. Implantable devices called deep brain stimulators can send electrical impulses to the area of the brain that is malfunctioning, stopping tremors and improving coordination. Other treatments include healthy lifestyle changes like adding in regular exercise, and eating a diet that includes plenty of vitamins C, D, and E.

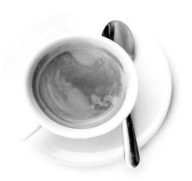

According to an article from the *Annals of Neurology*, never having smoked a cigarette and never drinking coffee or tea may slightly increase a person's risk in developing Parkinson's disease.

How Marijuana Can Help

For decades—centuries, even—people with Parkinson's have been praising cannabis for its ability to reduce tremors. Doctors all the way back in the nineteenth century used to prescribe cannabis tinctures to their patients with uncontrollable trembling, and now modern-day studies are backing up the practice. Research is showing that the cannabinoids in marijuana can improve the coordination and motor abilities of those with Parkinson's by binding with CB1 receptors in the brain. Other studies have found that the neuroprotective properties of cannabis may help prevent brain cells from dying and prevent the buildup of neurotoxins which contribute to the disease. Fox swears by CBD oil with no THC, as THC can affect mood and thinking. However, for those who also suffer from pain or muscle spasms, or from nausea as a side effect of other medications, a strain that includes THC may be helpful.

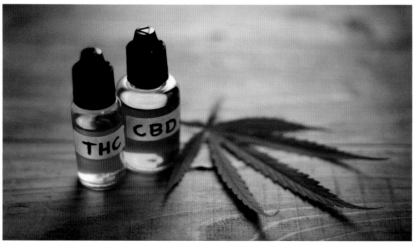

Oils, tinctures, and edibles make consumption of the drug easy for those with tremors and uncontrollable muscle movements.

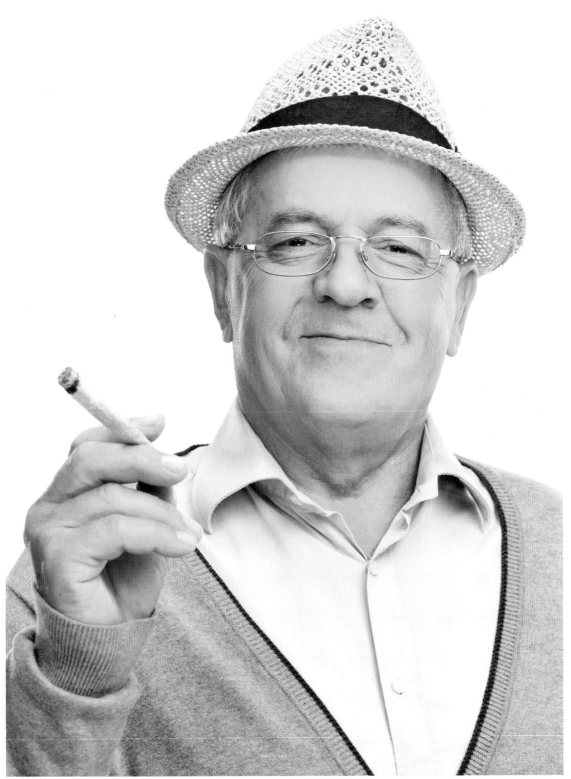

CTE

If you're a football fan, you've probably heard a lot about chronic traumatic encephalopathy, or CTE, in the news lately. This progressive, degenerative brain disorder—which can cause symptoms of memory loss, confusion, aggression, impaired judgment, anxiety, depression, and suicidal tendencies—is thought to have played a part in the behaviors of some of the NFL's most celebrated players. Perhaps the most famous was the case of New England Patriots player Aaron Hernandez, who was found guilty of murdering Odin Lloyd and later hanged himself in his prison cell. An autopsy discovered that the former NFL star had CTE—many believe it may have played a part in his aggressive temper and subsequent suicide.

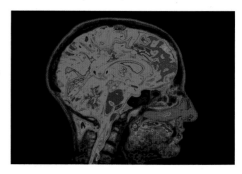

The only way to diagnose CTE is by looking at the tissue of the brain after death. The lack of recognized biomarkers while the patient is still alive leads to no conclusive answer of whether the patient may be suffering from CTE or not.

But Hernandez is far from the only athlete to have the disorder. Now, with 3.8 million sports-related concussions occurring every year in the U.S., CTE has gone from a little-known side effect of boxing to a serious—and possibly life-or-death—concern. One study found that up to eighty-seven percent of football players—whether playing in high school, college, or professionally—could be at risk of the disease.

Symptoms of CTE

The symptoms of CTE can begin years—or even decades—after the last brain trauma, so even if an athlete seems perfectly healthy when they end a career, there is no guarantee that symptoms won't show up down the road. Sadly, there is no specific treatment for the disorder, so patients must rely on treating each individual symptom—such as depression or anxiety—individually. While professional athletes may get all the publicity regarding CTE, the disorder is also common in military veterans, who may suffer repeated blows during training or in combat. Someone who is suffering from CTE might exhibit signs of ADHD, confusion, disorientation, dizziness, dementia, memory loss, speech impediments, tremors, vertigo, impulsive behavior.

Football has come under heavy scrutiny since 2008 because of the correlation found between the sports high-energy contact and the risk of developing CTE amongst its players. A 2013 study by the Boston University School of Medicine found that thirty-three of thirty-four football players tested port-mortem displayed definitive signs of CTE. A 2017 study by the *Journal of the American Medical Association* found that 110 of 111 brains of deceased football players showed clear signs of CTE.

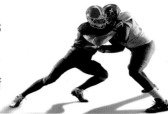

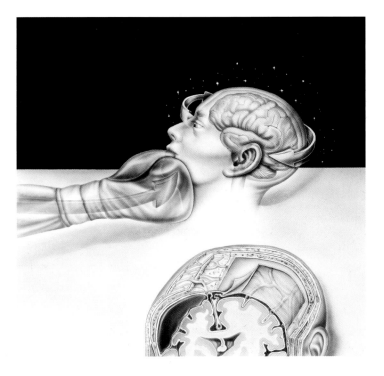

CTE is thought to be caused by repetitive head trauma, such as the frequent concussions suffered by football players or the head blows sustained by boxers. In fact, the disorder was first noticed in boxers back in the 1920s, when it was dubbed "punch drunk syndrome."

How Marijuana Can Help

There may be some hope in the form of medicinal cannabis. With CTE, inflammation in the brain causes a protein called Tau to form clumps, which slowly spread and kill off brain cells. Cannabis has been shown to increase blood flow to damaged areas of the brain, potentially warding off further damage and keeping tissue healthy. It is also known to have neuroprotective properties—the THC and CBD in marijuana have both been shown to reduce levels of toxins in the brain, as well as provide anti-inflammatory effects. And of course, cannabis has been shown to be effective in relieving many of CTE's symptoms, such as depression and mood changes.

Researchers are now looking into way that CBD—which is no longer banned by the World Anti-Doping Agency—could be used as a neuroprotective for everyone from service members heading into combat to boxers heading into the ring. The hope is that one day, those who are at risk for CTE can simply pop a pill designed to protect their brains from damage. But for now, the best way to prevent CTE is to avoid brain injury altogether. The NFL, for instance, is focusing on updating an outdated helmet design to better protect its players from head injuries. But those who are already suffering from the effects of CTE can still find relief from some of their symptoms by consuming cannabis in any number of ways. And hopefully, at the same time, they can slow the progression of this damaging disease.

Hope for Autism?

Around the world, about one percent of children are affected with autism spectrum disorder. This disorder encompasses four different diagnoses—autistic disorder, childhood disintegrative disorder, pervasive developmental disorder-not otherwise specified (PDD-NOS) and Asperger syndrome—all of which can cause varying degrees of communication difficulties, challenges with social skills, hypersensitivities to sound or light, or repetitive behaviors

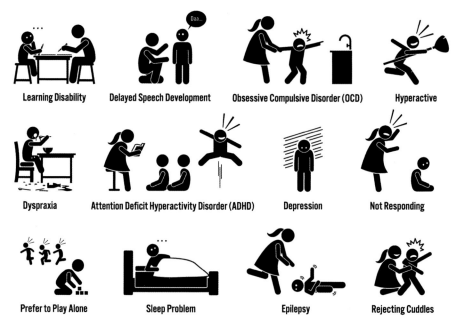

Learning Disability	Delayed Speech Development	Obsessive Compulsive Disorder (OCD)	Hyperactive
Dyspraxia	Attention Deficit Hyperactivity Disorder (ADHD)	Depression	Not Responding
Prefer to Play Alone	Sleep Problem	Epilepsy	Rejecting Cuddles

Symptoms of Autism

For some, the disorder can be mild, resulting in an impaired ability to read social cues, difficulty making friends, and discomfort with eye contact; but many of these children grow up to have fulfilling lives, albeit with challenges. But for others, autism is much more severe: For these children, symptoms can turn harmful or violent, and include repetitive head-banging, uncontrollable tantrums and rages, insomnia, and often an inability to speak. About one third of children with autism remain nonverbal throughout their lives.

Children with autism are also prone to other medical or mental health conditions, such as ADHD, anxiety disorders, gastrointestinal disorders, seizures, and phobias. Autism has no cure, so most treatments focus on these individual symptoms. Antianxiety or antipsychotic medications may be given, as well as ADHD drugs like Ritalin. For many children, these drugs only have an effect for a few hours; after that, symptoms can become even more extreme.

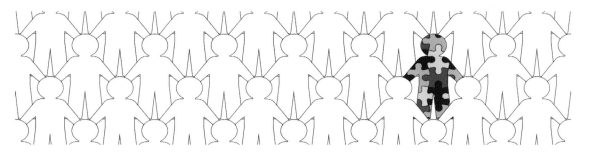

Autism disproportionately affects children in developed countries, with about one in fifty-nine children in the United States diagnosed with the disorder.

How Can Marijuana Help?

But what if there was a better treatment for autism? According to proponents of medicinal marijuana, there is. In fact, *Newsweek* magazine recently called cannabis "the world's most effective treatment for autism." Researchers took note of the success that cannabis had on children with severe epilepsy, and wondered if the drug's cannabinoids—which, as we know, have been shown to fight psychosis, depression, and anxiety—could have the same calming effect on those with autism.

An Israeli study of sixty autistic children showed that when given cannabis oil with a 20:1 ratio of CBD to THC, most children experienced a reduction in symptoms. Half of them had a significant reduction in symptoms, and a third of the children began speaking for the very first time. Studies like this have encouraged other parents of severely autistic children to set aside their preconceived notions of marijuana and see what the drug can offer. The anecdotal evidence has been extremely promising: Some children have had such a reduction in violent and disruptive symptoms that they've been able to move from special-needs school classes to standard classes. And parents of these children have found a hope they barely thought possible.

AUTISM

Unfortunately, as of 2018, only four states—Georgia, Minnesota, Oregon and Pennsylvania—include autism in their medicinal cannabis coverage. But as the evidence of marijuana's effectiveness for autism mounts and studies continue to offer positive outcomes, an FDA-approved cannabis treatment for children with autism may not be far off.

The causes of autism are still disputed, but there is strong evidence of genetic factors playing a role in diagnosis. The common worry that vaccinating children has a role in causing autism is largely disproven. Parents usually begin to notice signs of autism around the same time a child would begin to get vaccinated, causing a false correlation in the minds of parents.

Substance Abuse

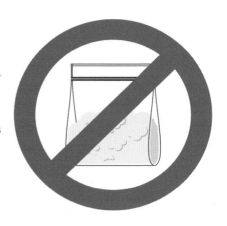

Of all the diseases, disorders, and conditions we've seen that may respond to treatment with medicinal cannabis, there is one that might seem out of place: the issue of substance abuse. In fact, the idea that marijuana is an illicit drug is so ingrained in our culture that the idea of using it to *fight* substance abuse seems like an oxymoron. But there is growing evidence that cannabis can help addicts walk away from substances that interfere with their quality of life.

This means that substance abuse is more than just a bad habit. People can develop a physical, as well as a psychological, dependence on certain drugs, and may also be genetically predisposed to addiction. The unpleasant symptoms that can occur when withdrawing from a substance—such as nausea and vomiting, anxiety, depression, hallucinations, and seizures—can last for days, or even weeks, and are often perceived as worse than continuing to take the drug itself.

Regardless of how or why it came about, ending the addiction is of utmost importance. Every year, around 90,000 Americans die as a result of drug or alcohol abuse, and the issue of addiction costs a staggering $700 billion in health care costs, lost productivity, and crime.

Sociocultural issues also influence addiction, with factors like income level, education, race, and age all having an effect on the likelihood of a person developing a dependence on a drug. And psychological issues, such as learned behaviors and influences at home, can also have an impact on the role of drug addiction in someone's life.

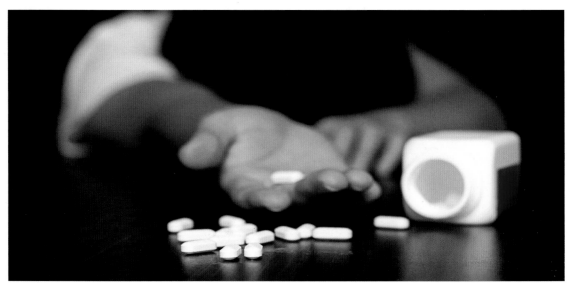

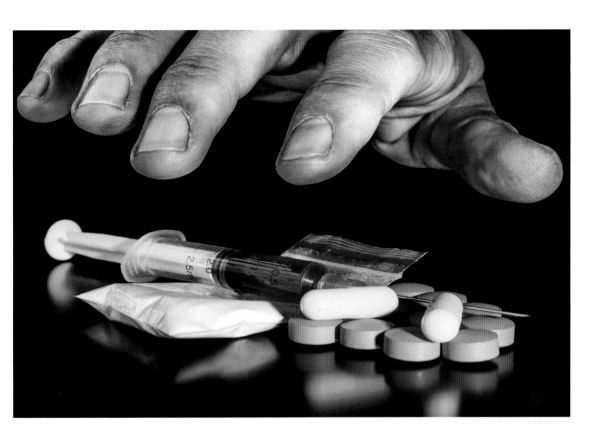

What Is Substance Abuse?

Simply stated, substance abuse is the chronic use of hazardous or damaging substances. The National Institute on Drug Abuse considers it a "relapsing brain disease that is characterized by compulsive drug seeking and use, despite harmful consequences." While an initial sampling of a drug is almost always a willing choice, once someone is within the throes of addiction their ability to make sound decisions becomes impaired. In fact, drug use physically changes areas of the brain responsible for judgment, learning, memory, and self-control.

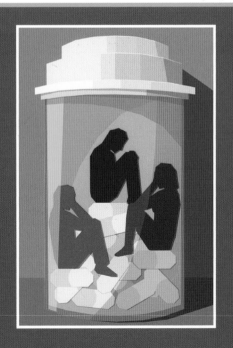

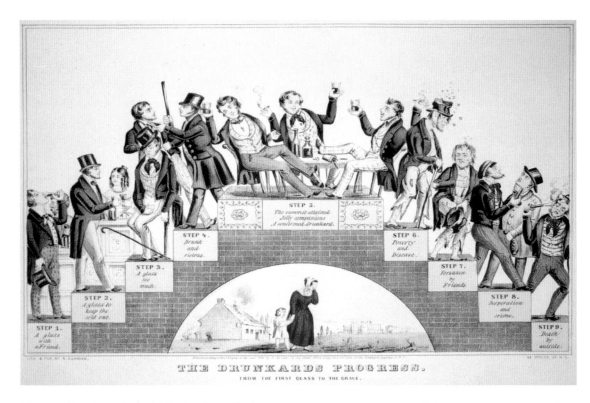

A lithographic print by Nathaniel Currier circa 1846 that was made to promote the cause of the temperance movement. It shows the purported descent that alcoholism leads its victims down. Step 1: A Glass With a Friend, Step 2: A Glass to Keep the Cold Out, Step 3: A Glass too Much, Step 4: Drunk and Riotous, Step 5: Jolly Companions and a Confirmed Drunk, Step 6: Poverty and Disease, Step 7: Forsaken by Friends, Step 8: Desperation and Crime, Step 9: Death by Suicide.

How Can Marijuana Help?

We've already seen how cannabis can be useful for reducing opioid use, which is one step towards fighting addiction. But studies are now finding that the cannabinoids in marijuana—especially non-psychoactive CBD—may help as a therapy for addiction. The CBD in cannabis, which provides a mood boost and relaxation without the "high," has been shown to ease anxiety and impulsiveness in those who are addicted to cocaine or alcohol, making it easier to avoid the substances.

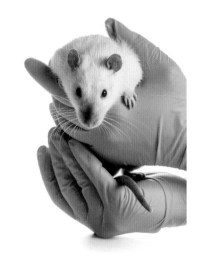

> Research in rodents has found that even small doses of cannabis are able to break heroin addiction in the animals—this could be a promising weapon in the fight against this highly addictive drug.

While some still view marijuana as an addictive substance itself, there are many who admit that the plant—even when it contains psychoactive THC—is not as dangerous or addictive as many other drugs. This makes it a popular choice for a "harms reduction" plan of attack towards substance abuse. Many who are addicted to drugs or alcohol find a "cold turkey" approach to quitting an unbearable option. By introducing cannabis in place of another substance, it becomes easier to let the other addiction go. This method is controversial, as some see this as simply replacing one addiction with another; but cannabis has a well-documented safety record compared to other drugs, as well as an extremely low risk of overdose. And while it is possible to become addicted to marijuana, only about 9 percent of users experience this; and breaking the addiction is much easier than giving up other drugs.

It's easy to see why this plant deserves to be taken into consideration when searching for alternative treatments. So many people suffering from so many issues have found relief with cannabis. Perhaps it's time we stopped thinking of it as a "bad" drug and start embracing its therapeutic properties. After all, most of us pop pills without a second thought any time we have a headache or strain a muscle—what if we're missing out on a more effective remedy just because of long-held stigmas and irrational stereotypes?

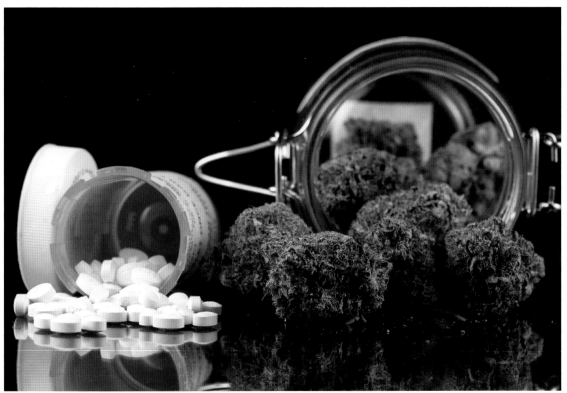

Cats, Canines, and Cannabis

Even if you're already familiar with the many medicinal benefits cannabis has to offer, you may not realize that the same benefits could help improve the lives of your four-legged friends. Just like humans, cats and dogs can suffer from a host of ailments and illnesses—arthritis, anxiety, nausea, irritable bowel syndrome, and cancer, just to name a few. For many of us, our pets are like family; but finding the best and most effective treatments for our furry family members isn't always easy. More and more pet parents are discovering that cannabis may be just the remedy they're searching for.

Helping Your Animal Friend

An increasing number of pet owners have found that the cannabinoids in these CBD and hemp products work wonders to help their suffering pets. Cannabis has been found to ease arthritis pain, calm anxiety and itching, lessen the frequency of seizures, and reduce noise phobias in dogs and cats. There have even been instances of cancer tumors shrinking in animals taking CBD, sometimes helping the pet go into complete remission. The drug works because just like humans, dogs and cats have an endocannabinoid system that helps to regulate processes like pain and mood. If cannabis is good enough for us humans, why shouldn't it also provide some of the same medicinal benefits to our pets?

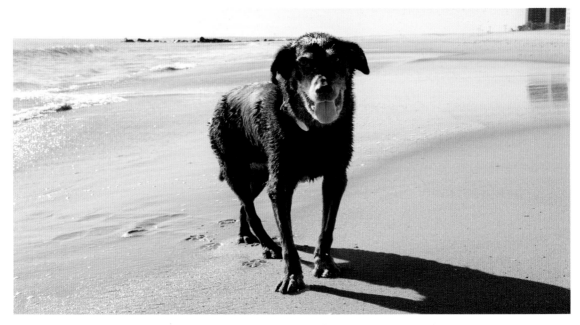

Many dogs will become arthritic as they age, and many owners will not notice the symptoms until the changes in the joints are severe. There are many supplements you can add to your dog's diet in order to reduce inflammation and help repair joints like glucosamine, omega-3 fatty acids, vitamin E, selenium, and methylsulfonylmethane. CBD oils can be very good to treat pain if you do not want to use prescription pain killers.

Unfortunately, veterinarians are prohibited from prescribing—and sometimes even recommending—cannabis for animals, so even if you live in a state where medicinal marijuana is legal, it's impossible to procure a medical cannabis card for your pet. But the good news is, CBD and hemp products are widely available online, and many are now specifically formulated for pets. While there has been little formal research into the effects of CBD and hemp on dogs and cats, those who have tried it for their furry family members have found great success. In fact, researchers consider pets to be the perfect subjects for attesting to the efficacy of CBD and hemp. Since animals don't understand what you're giving them, there can be no placebo effect. Therefore, if cannabis works for a pet, it works! Still, it is a good idea to talk to your vet before giving your pet a CBD or hemp product, and to always be careful with the dosage: Dogs are ten times more sensitive to THC than humans, so even trace amounts of it in a CBD product can cause side effects.

As humans continue to discover medicinal uses for the cannabis plant, its popularity grows. And with that popularity comes benefits not just for us, but for our four-legged companions, as well.

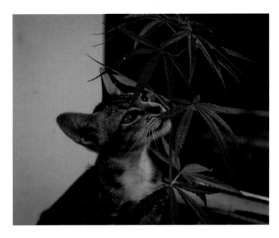

Cats are notorious for being a bit too curious. You may find that your cat is attracted to the smell of your dried cannabis or even live plants, which can lead to the cat nibbling on something that it should not be nibbling on. Uncoordinated movement, fickle moods, vomiting, slow heart rate, and seizures can all be signs that your cat was exposed to marijuana.

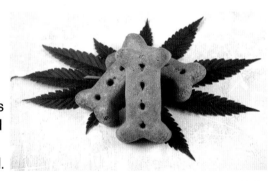

Biscuits, chews, treats, and supplements can be added to your pet's diet, or you can try an oil or tincture.

How Marijuana Can Help

While pets and humans may have some of the same symptoms—and, therefore, the same reasons to consume medicinal marijuana—the way each species is affected by cannabis is different. The THC in the drug may simply provide a pleasant "high" for a human, and overdosing is nearly impossible; however, for animals, THC can have toxic side effects, and an overdose can be fatal in rare cases. For this reason, it is recommended that pet owners stick to products that contain very little (if any) THC. Many people have found that giving their pet companions CBD or hemp products is the best way to avoid any dangerous side effects.

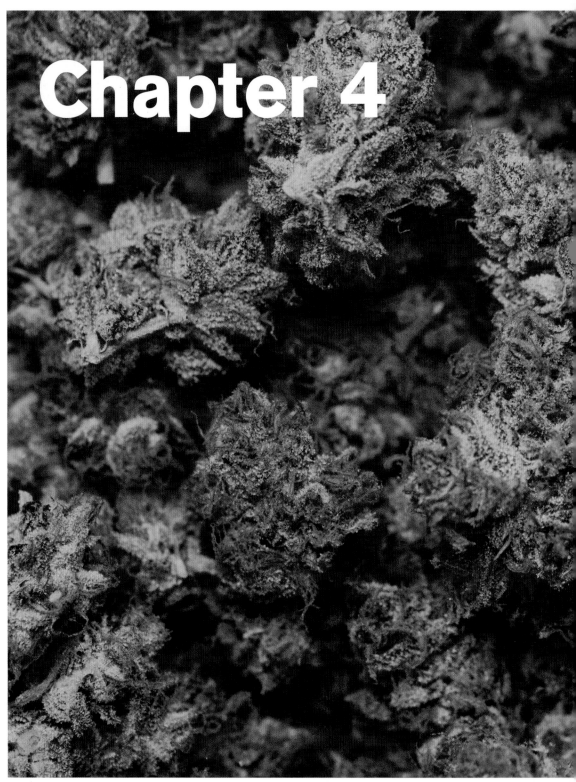

Chapter 4

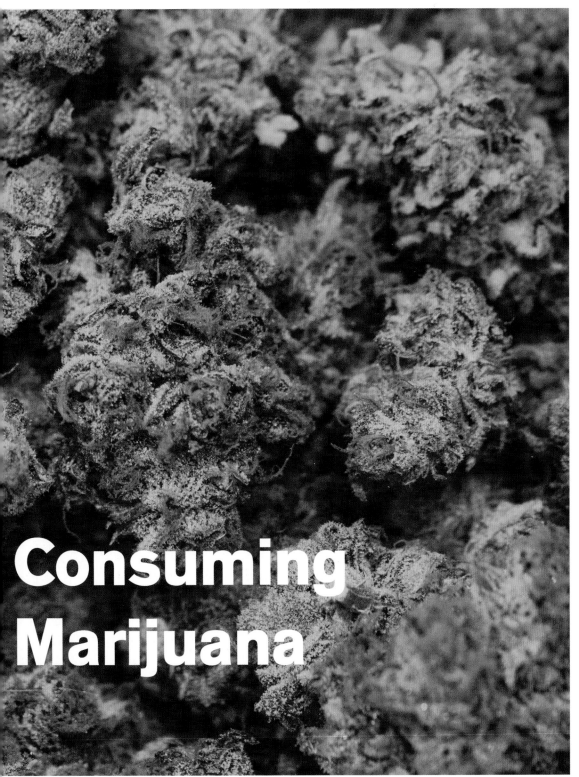

Consuming Marijuana

Lighting Up

For many of us, the image of a "stoner" rolling a joint and puffing away has pretty much been our only idea of what it's like to ingest cannabis. Movies like *Dazed and Confused* and *Harold and Kumar Go to White Castle* serve to perpetuate this idea, while creating characters who seem a bit lazy, befuddled, or downright stupid. It's enough to make anyone think twice before delving into the world of cannabis. But if we set aside our preconceived notions, we'll discover there's much more to the plant than the movies would have us believe. And you don't need to be a "stoner"—or even smoke—to reap the benefits. The more popular the drug becomes, the more ways its proponents devise to consume it.

Of course, some people who ingest cannabis do still choose to smoke the drug, and there's good reason for this: Marijuana that is smoked takes a quick, direct route to the brain. This means that the effects are felt extremely quickly. Smoking makes it very easy to tell when "enough is enough," so once the desired effect is reached, the user can stop before feeling any unwanted side effects. This method can be useful when feeling relief from an ailment just can't come quickly enough—like severe nausea or vomiting.

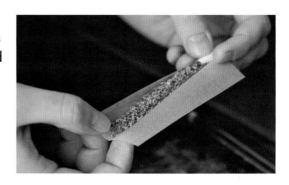

Although it may be difficult to first learn how to roll a joint, they are a very effective and enjoyable way to smoke marijuana.

Possible Drawbacks

Smoking does have drawbacks, however. It is, after all, *smoking*—that thing that we've all been cautioned against for most of our lives. And while the effects of marijuana smoke on the lungs have not been extensively studied, most experts agree that inhaling any kind of combustible material on a regular basis can irritate and inflame the respiratory tract. The effects of smoking also don't last as long as some other ingestion methods. But when a fast-acting remedy is the priority, smoking is a top choice.

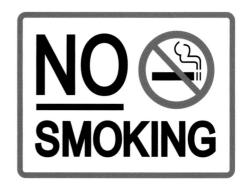

Heavily and chronically smoking marijuana can cause coughing, production of sputum, wheezing, and chronic bronchitis. The tar of cannabis smoke is chemically similar to that of tobacco smoke, containing dozens of known carcinogens.

What Are You Smoking?

The buds of the cannabis plant are the most common part that is used to smoke, because they contain a high concentration of cannabinoids. Flowers are popular to smoke, as well, especially since this is where the cannabinoid-packed trichomes are located. Most smokers avoid the leaves of the plant, since the effects, if any, are negligible.

Kief and hash can also be smoked—many users simply add a bit of either substance over cannabis buds or flowers, or just regular tobacco, to add an extra "kick." The same can be done with oils and other concentrates, although it's not a favorite method amongst cannabis connoisseurs as it doesn't provide a chance to experience the potency of the concentrate on its own. But all of these can also be smoked on their own.

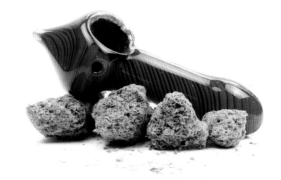

It is true that you can make your own pipes and devices at home to smoke marijuana, but it is highly recommended you visit your local head shop to buy an actual pipe to use.

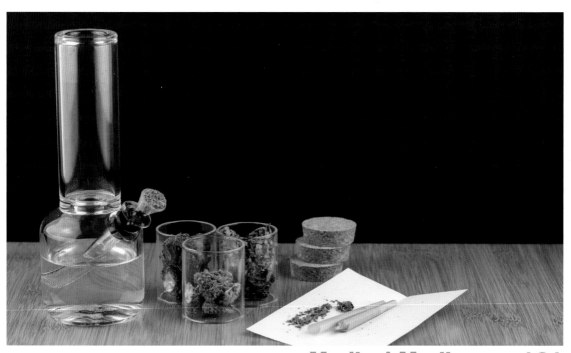

Stick That in Your Pipe and Smoke It

Not only are there a multitude of different ways to consume cannabis, but there are also several different ways just to smoke it. We're all familiar with the idea of a "joint," or doobie. This, of course, is a hand-rolled marijuana cigarette. To make the process easy, joint rolling kits are available that include everything you need to roll the perfect cannabis cigarette.

Rolling experts recommend using a "crutch," or a filtered rolling tip, to make rolling the joint easier. This provides a pre-formed shape to work with, which the rolling paper can wrap around. After evenly distributing your cannabis product into the paper, the joint can then be rolled into a "pinner"—a thin, traditional cigarette shape—or a cone shape. Pre-made cones are also available for those who have trouble rolling their own joints.

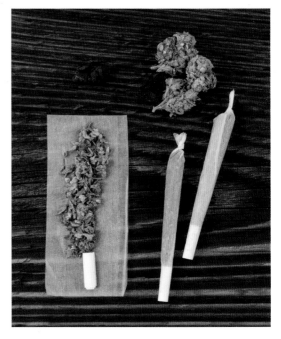

Marijuana must be processed in order for the joint to burn all the way through.

Pipes

Pipes are another option. Adapted from traditional tobacco pipes, cannabis pipes are usually made of glass, with a bowl on one end to hold marijuana, and a tube through which smoke can be inhaled. Once cannabis is packed into the bowl, it is heated with a lighter, a wick, or a glass wand that is warmed to the point where it will vaporize the cannabis. Pipe screens are also available that may be used in the bowl of the pipe to prevent inhalation of burning bits of cannabis.

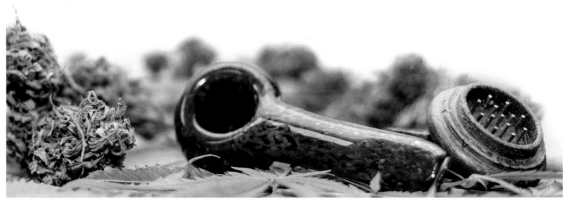

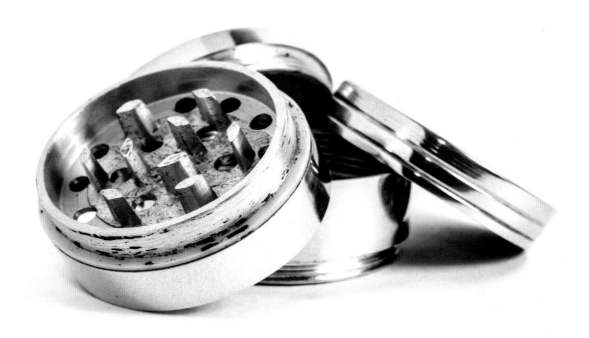

Marijuana must be processed in order for the joint to burn all the way through.

How to Take a Hit Off of a Glass Pipe

A glass pipe is different from a straight pipe in that it does not provide a direct channel of inhalation. Between the bowl (where you load the ground marijuana) and the mouthpiece (where you inhale the smoke from) is the chamber that fills with smoke as you pull (inhale through) the pipe. While pulling, you'll want to cover the carb (the hole on the side of the pipe) with a finger, let the chamber fill with smoke, and then release your finger to inhale all of the smoke from the chamber. You can alternate the intervals between releasing and covering the carb to take larger or smaller hits. You can even release and cover the carb multiple times in one inhalation.

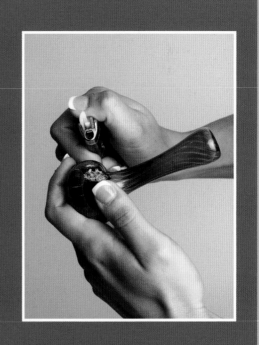

Straight Pipes

Another way to smoke cannabis is with a "chillum," or a straight pipe. Chillums have been around since at least the eighteenth century, when they were used by Hindu monks in India. Traditionally, the pipes were made of clay, but nowadays you can usually find them made of glass, sometimes fashioned into whimsical shapes like fish, mushrooms, or flutes.

Using the same kind of straight-pipe method are "one hitters," which, as the name suggests, are designed to hold a very small amount of cannabis—enough for "one hit." Chillums and one hitters are generally convenient and discreet—some decorative chillums can even be worn around the neck as a pendant when not in use.

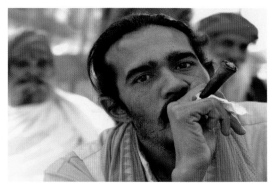

A Hindu devotee smoking from a traditional chillum.

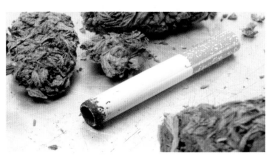

This straight pipe that looks like a cigarette is known as a bat, or one-hitter. Bats can be used in conjunction with dugout boxes. Dugout boxes provide you with a compact container that will neatly hold ground marijuana and your one hitter.

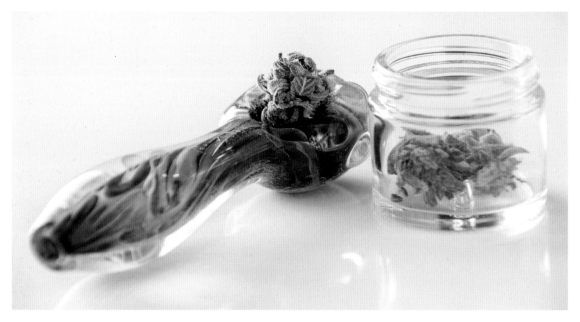

Hand blown glass pipes can be very unique in design, color, and size. Some can even change colors after use.

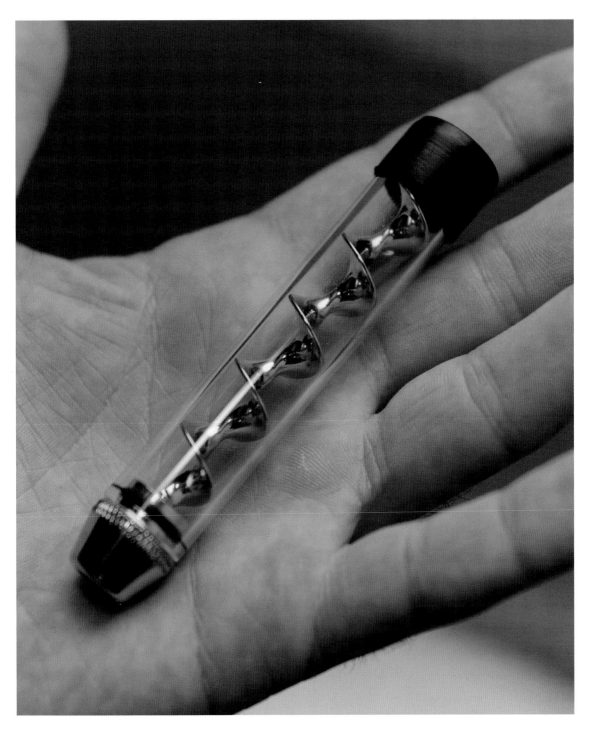

Glass blunt tubes can be filled with ground cannabis and smoked like a cigar. The spiral screw-like center is used to push the marijuana to the front of the pipe, and at the same time push the ash out.

Bongs and Bubblers

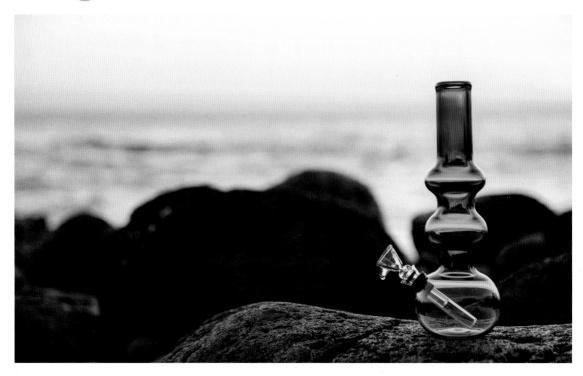

Water pipes, like bongs and bubblers (which are just mini bongs) are one of the most popular ways to consume cannabis. With bongs, smoke from the marijuana is circulated and filtered through water before inhalation. The method has been used for millennia—tales of bongs can be traced back to China's Ming Dynasty and ancient Africa and Asia; archeologists even recently discovered two 2,400-year-old solid gold bongs near the Caucasus Mountains!

The Lowdown on Bongs

Today, bongs are rarely quite so extravagant as the solid-gold bongs of yore, usually made of hand-blown glass. They are made up of certain basic parts: The bowl, where cannabis is placed; the downstem, a small tube that allows smoke to travel down into the water; the base, which can take many different shapes including beakers, cylinders, and bulbs; and the tube, which is what fills with smoke after it has filtered through the water.

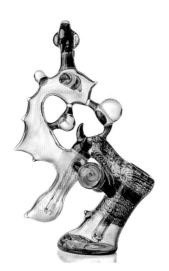

This custom-blown bubbler is very pretty, but it could be very difficult to clean when the time comes.

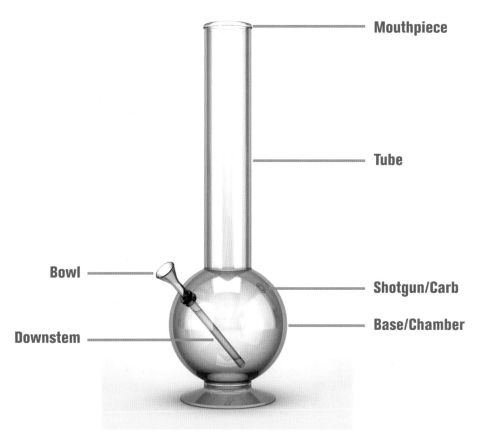

Mouthpiece

Tube

Bowl

Shotgun/Carb

Base/Chamber

Downstem

This is a standard bong with a bulbous base and regular downstem. There are many accessories you can buy for your bong that will make it smoother to smoke if the factory setup is too harsh.

Percolators

Percolators are used as extra filtration stages in the smoking process. The main purpose for their use is to a create a smoother hit by purifying and cooling down the smoke. There are many different styles of percolators including the coil (seen here), honeycomb, tree, inline, matrix, turbine, showerhead, and more. It can be awfully confusing wrapping your head around the vast technology that is used for bongs, but your local head shop employee should be able to answer all of your questions and help you find what is right for you.

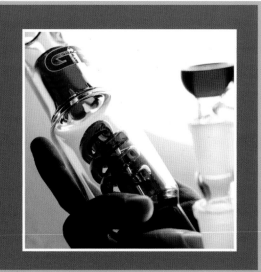

Although most bongs will have detachable or sliding downstems you can use to pull out to clear the smoke from the bong's chamber, some bongs, like this one, will feature a carb on the side of the base that you must cover and release to inhale the smoke.

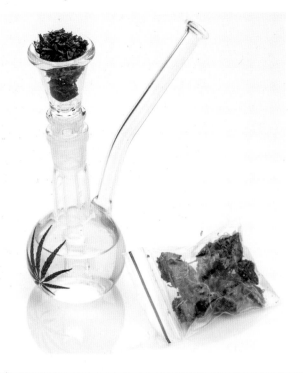

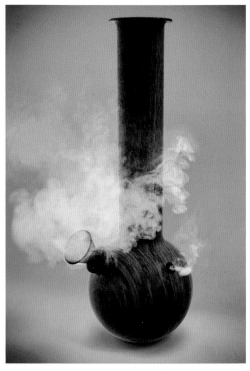

Bubblers can come with built in down stems or they can have detachable downstems like the one seen in this photo.

Diffusers

Most downstems only provide one opening for the smoke to be percolated and filtered through the water, but diffused downstems have multiple openings at the bottom of the downstem to spread the smoke more evenly through the filtration medium, cooling and smoothing out the smoke for a better hit.

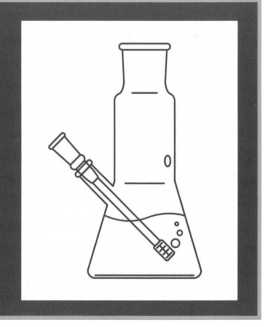

The Benefits of Bongs

Many users prefer bongs over other methods of smoking, because the smoke is filtered and cooled before it is inhaled. This can be easier on the throat and lungs than the hotter, drier heat that is experienced with joints or pipes. And bubblers provide the convenience of a smaller pipe, while still offering filtered smoke. However, their smaller parts can have a tendency to get clogged, so it's important to regularly clean bubblers.

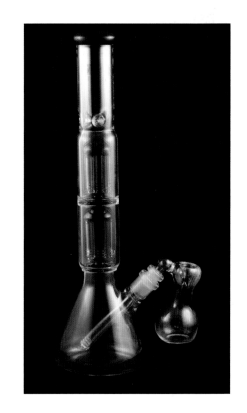

This bong has many added features that amount to a more pleasant and less harsh smoking experience. The bowl has an ash catcher that filters debris before it reaches the main chamber's water. The downstem has also been upgraded to a glass-on-glass diffused downstem. Working up the tube from the base, there are two four-armed tree percolators all with diffused downstems. In the section before the mouthpiece there is a place in which you can put ice to cool down the smoke. This bong would provide a very clean smoking experience with its four stages of water filtration.

Cleaning Your Bongs and Bubblers

You will want to refresh the water in your bong and bubbler after every use because it can get awfully nasty from the ash and other impurities it filters from the smoke. After prolonged use of the same water, a smell can emerge from your pipe that can really hamper the pleasures of your smoking experience. Bong water is nothing you want to mess with! The glass itself of the pipe can also become caked with resinous material that is very difficult to manage. There are a variety of pipe cleaning solutions you can use that will get the job done, like Formula 420, Grunge Off, or Orange Chronic. Use bottle or tube brushes to scrub harder to reach areas of your pipe. Pipe cleaners are good for clearing out your downstem and bowl as well.

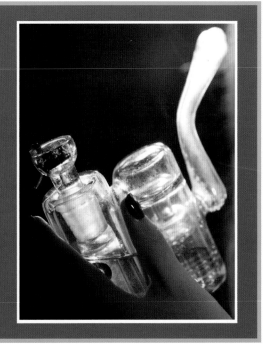

Dabs

If none of these other smoking methods resonates, there's still one option left: dabbing. Dabbing is a method to smoke cannabis concentrates, like waxes and oils. Using a water pipe called a "dab rig," a concentrate is placed onto a heated attachment called a "nail" or "banger" where it is vaporized and then inhaled. Dab rigs can be purchased specifically for this purpose, or a regular water pipe can be used with dabbing attachments. Unlike the time-tested bong, dabbing has only been around for about a decade; but with more and more cannabis concentrates hitting the market, the method is growing in popularity, so new attachments and accessories are becoming available all the time.

Because dabbing uses concentrates, this method produces very fast—and sometimes very powerful—effects. So it's best to start with an extremely small amount of concentrate—no bigger than a crumb. While it may take some trial and error to find the correct amount of concentrate to use, those who suffer from chronic pain or nausea often say that dabbing is one of the best ways to bring swift relief from their symptoms. Concentrates also eliminate the resin and smoke that result from burning plant matter, making the method easier on the lungs. And if you're looking for the therapeutic effects of cannabinoids without the "high," nonintoxicating CBD concentrates can also be dabbed.

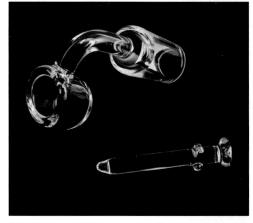

A quartz banger and a quartz nail.

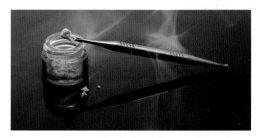

As opposed to smoking buds or flowers, you only need very small amounts of concentrate to reach the desired effect.

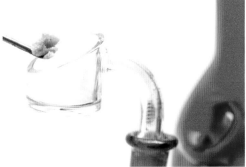

This device is called a quartz banger which attaches to the downstem of your bong or bubbler.

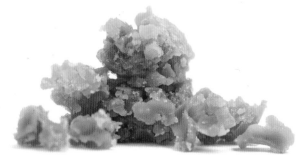

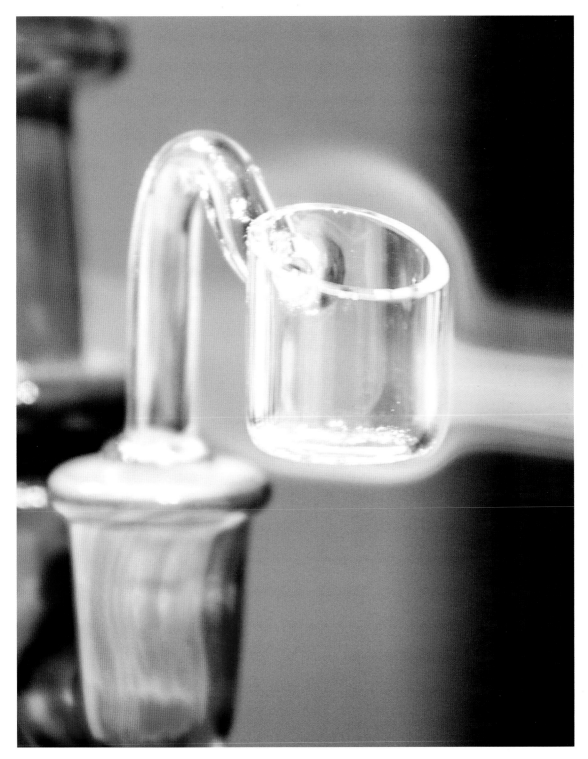

Before you put the wax in the banger, you heat the banger up with a torch lighter so that it will vaporize the wax upon contact.

Vaporized

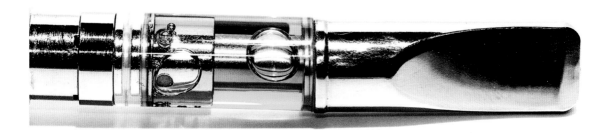

Although many experts agree that smoking marijuana doesn't carry as many risks as smoking cigarettes, it does still require inhaling carcinogenic tars and gases. And regular cannabis smokers are at greater risk of issues like bronchitis and respiratory infections. So if you'd rather avoid inhaling smoke altogether, a vaporization method may be just the thing you're looking for.

Benefits of Vaping

Vaporizing marijuana—or vaping—allows the user to inhale steam instead of smoke. By heating the cannabis to a point just before it burns—usually between 350 and 400 degrees Fahrenheit—it releases vapors which are packed with the same cannabinoids and benefits found when it is smoked, but without the irritating toxins.

Vaping has many benefits, as well. Like smoking, the effects of vaporized marijuana work quickly, making it a good choice for anyone who needs immediate relief from pain or nausea. Vaping also uses up to thirty percent less cannabis than would be used for smoking, so less marijuana goes to waste. Vaporizers come in several different sizes—from larger, stationary vaporizers for home use, to portable units about the size of a cell phone, to pen-sized vaporizers aptly named "vape pens." While larger and more unwieldy, stationary vaporizers tend to provide higher quality vapor and are equipped with stronger heating elements. But portable vaporizers and vape pens are popular with those who travel frequently or wish for something more discreet.

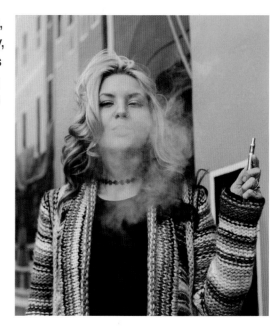

The vapor of vaping is not vapor at all, but aerosol.

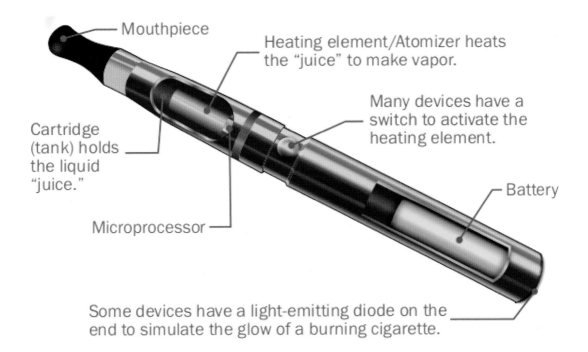

Mouthpiece

Heating element/Atomizer heats the "juice" to make vapor.

Many devices have a switch to activate the heating element.

Cartridge (tank) holds the liquid "juice."

Battery

Microprocessor

Some devices have a light-emitting diode on the end to simulate the glow of a burning cigarette.

Conduction and Convention

There are two different kinds of heat used in vaporizers—conduction and convection. Conduction heaters transfer heat directly from a heat source to the heated material, meaning the cannabis is in constant contact with the heat source. Vaporizers that use these heaters are less expensive, uncomplicated, and quick to warm up; but the temperature can be harder to control and the cannabis must be stirred to ensure even heating. Convection heaters pass hot air through the chamber that holds the cannabis, which heats more evenly and is easier to control. However, these vaporizers are more expensive and take longer to warm up.

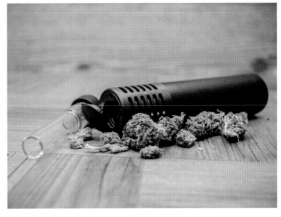

A study conducted by the University of California, San Francisco, found that vaping marijuana can reduce the amount of harmful combustion products that one is normally exposed to when smoking marijuana.

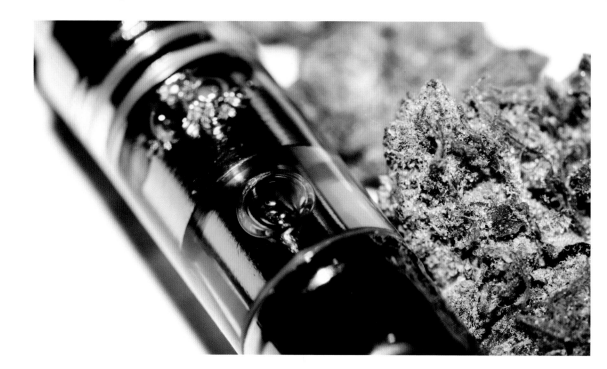

What Can You Vape?

If you can smoke it, you can also vape it—buds, flowers, oils, waxes, and concentrates can all be used in vaporizers. But the product you prefer may also dictate what type of vaporizer you should use. Many vapers feel that using the actual flowers and buds provides the best effects, and generally stationary or portable vaporizers work best for this. But vape pens are surging in popularity, which means that manufacturers have begun developing some pens that work with dry material. But for the most part, vape pens work best with oils and other concentrates.

While vaporizing can be a great choice for consuming cannabis, it does have its downsides, as well. When vaporizing dry cannabis, new users who are unfamiliar with their equipment may accidentally set the heat too high—which results in unusable, combusted cannabis. This can be especially difficult when using a vaporizer with a conduction heater. But the learning curve is generally short, and most vapers are quickly able to find the perfect vaporizing temperature for their particular setup. When vaping concentrates, care needs to be taken with the dosing, as waxes and oils tend to have a much higher percentage of THC than flowers or buds. Also, it should be noted that so far, no one regulates the ingredients that go into pre-filled vaping cartridges, and common additives like propylene glycol and polyethylene glycol may not be healthy to inhale.

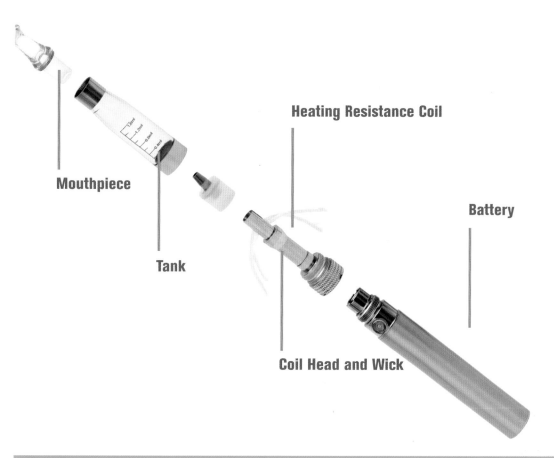

Mouthpiece

Tank

Heating Resistance Coil

Battery

Coil Head and Wick

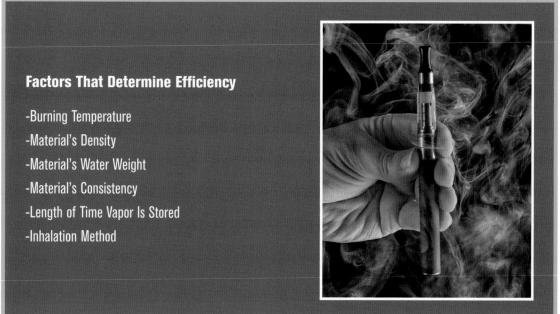

Factors That Determine Efficiency

-Burning Temperature

-Material's Density

-Material's Water Weight

-Material's Consistency

-Length of Time Vapor Is Stored

-Inhalation Method

Feeling Hungry?

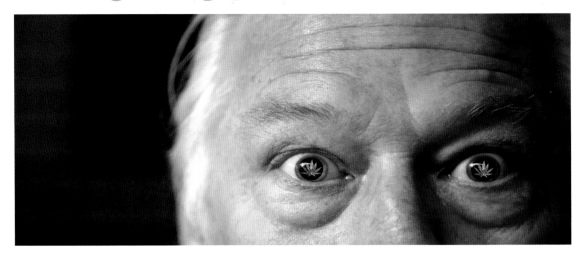

Eaten cannabis is said to produce more "body-centered" effects than smoking or vaping—the effects are more evenly distributed throughout the body.

If inhaling anything—whether it be smoke or vapor—still seems like a bad idea, don't fret: There are a few consumption methods left, and they may be the simplest methods of all. We're talking, of course, about edibles and topicals. One of the biggest benefits of using edibles as a consumption method is its convenience—what could be easier than simply chewing and swallowing? The effects of cannabis that has been eaten last much longer than other methods, as well: Smoked or vaped marijuana produces effects that last between one and three hours; whereas the effects of eaten marijuana can last up to seven hours. This can be a huge pro for someone seeking more than a temporary respite from unpleasant symptoms.

But as we've already discussed, the effects of eaten cannabis can take up to two hours to manifest. This may be too long to wait for someone who is suffering from an unbearable symptom. And of course, since it takes so long for eaten cannabis to kick in, it can be easy to accidentally ingest too much. It's always important to start with a small dose, and to wait until you feel the effects before taking any more.

What's on the Menu?

For those who wish to give edibles a try, there are a myriad of options to choose from. Sure, you can still find "pot brownies" to indulge a sweet tooth, but the world of cannabis edibles encompasses so much more. Cannabis-infused chocolate bars, cereals, ice cream, mints, and gummies are all widely available products, but savory snacks are on the market as well, like cheese puffs, beef jerky, pretzels, popcorn, and nuts. As you can see, there's something for everyone!

If you prefer to drink your dose of cannabis, no problem—the marijuana beverage market keeps growing. Try a soothing cup of cannabis tea, a cup of coffee, a fizzy soda, or a refreshing lemonade. Be sure to check the dosage, as these drinks come with anywhere from 10 mg to more than 150 mg of THC per bottle.

If you'd rather try your hand at making your own edibles, the internet is full of recipes for infused ingredients. Cannabis butter—or "cannabutter"—is wildly popular, because it can easily be added to dozens of recipes. Cookies, cakes, brownies, even pasta sauces can all get an extra "kick" from cannabutter. But don't stop with butter—you can infuse oil, milk, honey, and alcohol, or make a cannabis-infused simple syrup that can be added to drinks and smoothies.

How Much Should You Take?

With edibles, dosing is very important. Once you've eaten something, you can't avoid the effects it will bring, so you want to be sure you don't go overboard. Body mass, age, gender, and metabolism all play a role in how much cannabis you can ingest before feeling your desired effect, and everyone is different. Experts recommend treating edibles like you would any other painkiller or medicine—don't take it on an empty stomach. Even though the edible itself is food, make sure to eat something else (drug free) along with it. Most people consider 10 mg of THC to be one dose, so pay attention to serving sizes or the total amount of THC in your edible item. This may still require some trial and error, as you may find that a gummy with 10 mg of THC may affect you differently than the same amount in a chocolate or a drink. And of course, remember to wait at least an hour before making a decision to up the dosage.

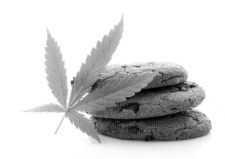

While edibles may be a great option for most people, they can pose another con for those with severe nausea or vomiting--the idea of eating anything, even something that may improve symptoms, can be impossible for someone with these conditions.

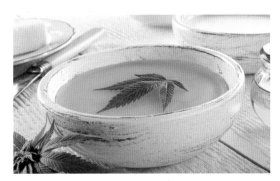

Cannabis butter is a relatively easy way you can begin to make your own marijuana edibles. After you have made the butter you can use your butter to replace all the butter your favorite recipe calls for.

More Than Skin Deep

Consuming cannabis can have amazing effects for a host of different issues, but you don't even have to ingest it to reap some of the benefits. Cannabis-infused topicals can help soothe arthritis, sports injuries, and burns—and they're non-psychoactive, so they can be used any time. These creams, oils, balms, and lotions bind with the CB2 receptors in your skin, immediately bringing localized relief to areas feeling painful or sore. And topically applied cannabis may even prevent skin from aging, as CBD has been found to be a more potent antioxidant than even vitamins C or E!

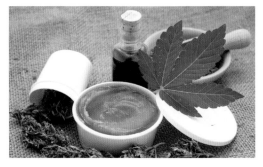

If you don't have a specific area on your body that is causing you pain at the moment, there are still many areas that can be messaged with topical marijuana ointments. Areas like the temples, knees, neck, wrists, shoulders, and feet are all overused body parts that could benefit from some relief.

Just like edibles, the topical cannabis market is continually expanding. You can find balms, lotions, bath salts, lip balms, oils, and more. The type of product you use may depend on the issue you're trying to address. For intense or localized pain, try a balm—they have a higher concentration of active ingredients and absorb quickly. Less intense or more general pain may benefit from a lotion, as these are easy to spread over large areas of skin and are not as concentrated as a balm. Oils are great for a soothing massage, or for areas with extra rough skin that may need relief. Bath salts are perfect to use before bed, as they can ease pain and promote restful sleep. And if you don't like any of the products on the market? Check the always-helpful internet for some simple do-it-yourself recipes for cannabis-infused lotions, oils, and creams.

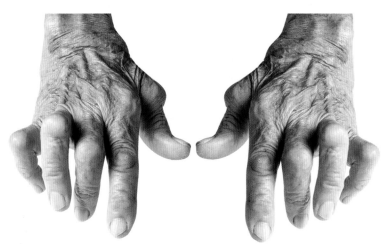

Marijuana topicals are really helpful for those with arthritis.

Cannabinoids have even been shown to have antibacterial properties, meaning you can use a topical to not only ease the pain of scratches, scrapes, and bug bites, but prevent infection, as well.

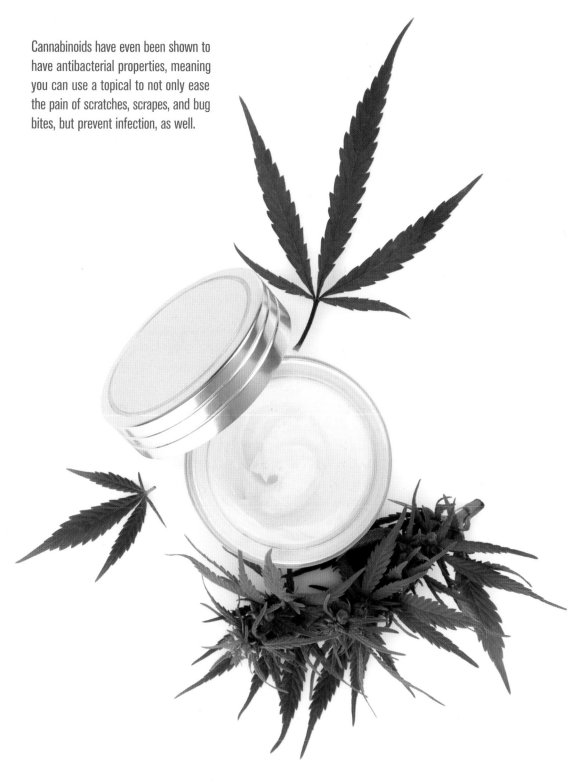

Green Medicine

We've seen quite an amazing list of marijuana's possibilities: From relieving chronic pain to stopping seizures to calming anxiety; from improving the quality of life of cancer patients to giving Alzheimer's patients hope; from breaking addictions to rediscovering the joys of life—there's so much more to this "weed" than we often admit. It's not just about high school kids secretly smoking behind the gym or Harold and Kumar's hunger-fueled search for hamburgers: This oft-satirized plant may hold the keys to countless medical advancements.

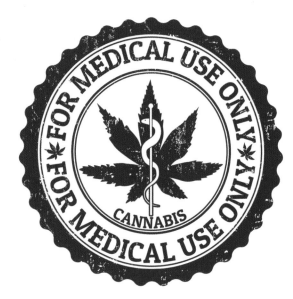

While the world of marijuana has come a long way since the days of tie-dyed hippies and Woodstock, stereotypes, myths, and assumptions still affect our thoughts and feelings about it. Hopefully, as we learn more about cannabis and the many benefits it may provide, we can think of it less as an illicit drug and more as a therapeutic treatment. Steps toward legalization still need to be taken, but with more and more people embracing its effects and an explosively expanding cannabis industry now in the U.S., it's hard to imagine the momentum will slow down any time soon. Perhaps the future of medicine will, indeed, be green.

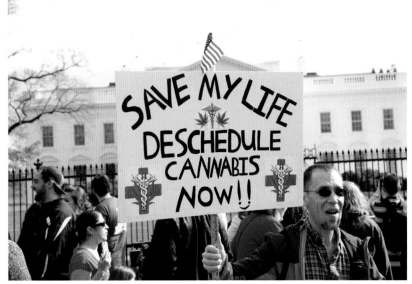

A protest outside of the White House on April 2, 2016 to reschedule marijuana. Protesters demonstrated and smoked pot outside of the White House that day to prove that the drug was not dangerous. According to an AP report covering that day's activities, many protesters and organizers saw former President Obama's pot policy to be hypocritical because of his admittance to smoking pot when he was younger.

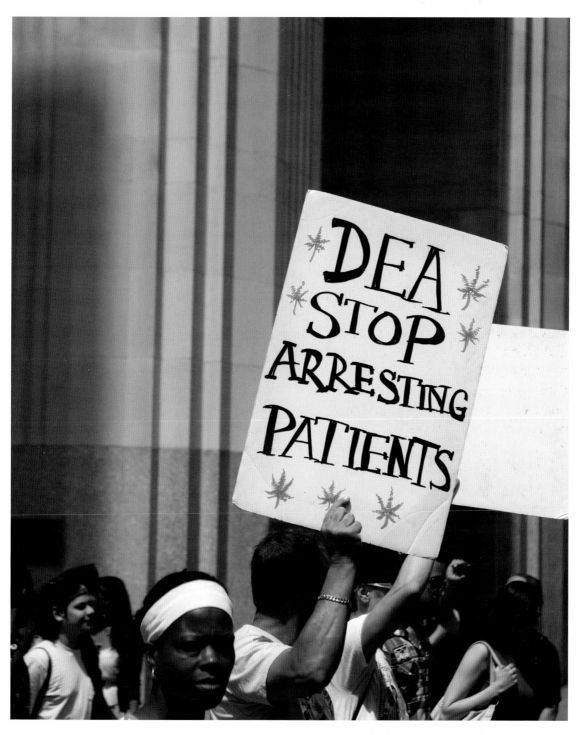

A protest in Mew York City on May 1, 2010. Organized protests against the illegal status of marijuana have been organized for decades around the world, but it seems that many advancements for the cause are being made in the twenty-tens.

Popular Medicinal Strains Index

AK–47 (Hybrid)

Characteristics:

This sativa dominant hybrid is a mix between Colombian, Mexican, Thai, and Afghani strains, creating a complex amalgamation of flavors and effects. First bred in 1992 by Serious Seeds, AK-47 has won multiple Cannabis Cup awards for its high percentages of THC.

Use For:

Stress, Depression, Lack of Appetite, Pain, Headaches

Effects:

Relaxed, Happy, Uplifted, Creative, Euphoric

Constituents:

14–20% THC

1.5% CBD

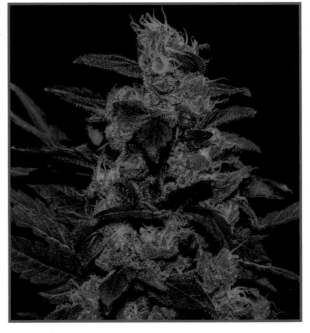

Berry Noir (Indica)

Characteristics:

This indica strain is a cross between Platinum OG, Blackberry, and Girl Scout Cookies. It was featured in the LA Medical Cannabis Cup in 2014 and is often thought to consist of high percentages of THC, but no tests have been done to take an actual measurement.

Use For:

Stress, Depression, Insomnia

Constituents:

Not Yet Measured

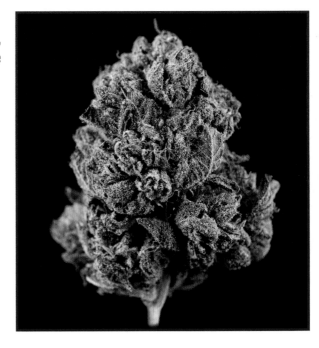

Blue Dream (Hybrid)

Characteristics:

Blue Dream, a sativa-leaning hybrid with a lineage of indica Blueberry and sativa Haze, has a berry aroma, an indica phenotype, and a high-THC concentration. It is mentally invigorating but also effective for pain relief without being highly sedative.

Use For:

Pain, Depression, Nausea, Fatigue, Lack of Appetite

Constituents:

17–24% THC

0.1-0.2% CBD

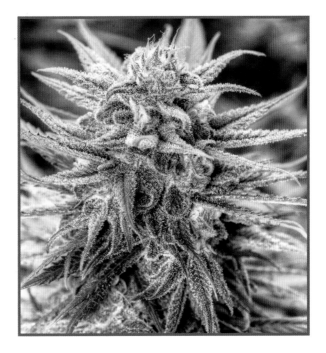

Durban Poison (Sativa)

Characteristics:

A very powerful, pure sativa strain from the South African city of Durban. It creates an energetic effect that will keep you productive with your creative or recreational activities. It has a sweet smell and has large resin glands that make Durban Poison an ideal strain for creating concentrates.

Use For:

Depression, Stress, Fatigue, Pain, Headaches

Effects:

Energetic, Uplifted, Happy, Euphoric, Focused

Constituents:

16–25% THC

0.2% CBD

0.6–1.4% CBG

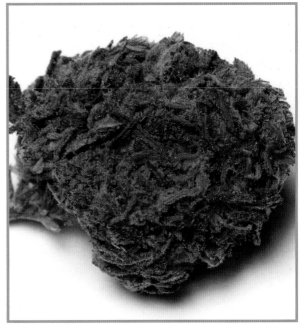

Golden Goat (Hybrid)

Characteristics:

This light-green, and often pink-tinged, strain was created by an accidental pollination of an Island Sweet Skunk by a Hawaiian-Romulan in Topeka, Kansas. Although it is a hybrid, it is sativa dominant with sweet, sour, and spicy aroma.

Use For:

Stress, Depression, Pain, Fatigue, Headaches

Effects:

Happy, Uplifted, Euphoric, Energetic, Relaxed

Constituents:

12–23% THC

0.06% CBD

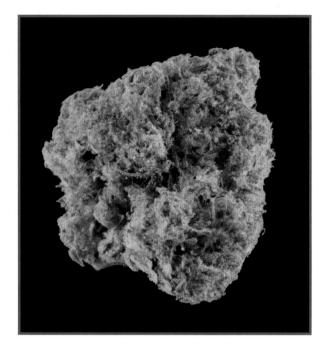

Grandaddy Purple (Indica)

Characteristics:

Debuting in 2003, Grandaddy Purple was spawned from the relaxing genetics of Purple Urkle and Big Bud indica strains. With an aroma reminiscent of grape and berry flavors and a deep purple color in its blooms, Grandaddy Purple is a vibrant strain that provides deep states of relaxation and euphoria.

Use For:

Stress, Pain, Insomnia, Depression

Effects:

Relaxed, Sleepy, Happy, Hungry

Constituents:

17–23% THC

0.1% CBD

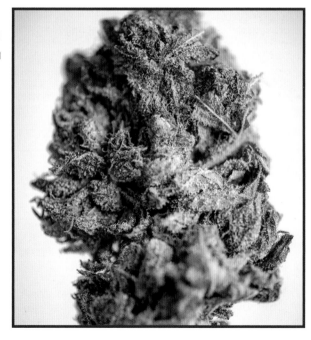

Grape Ape (Indica)

Characteristics:

Grape Ape was propagated by Apothecary Genetics and Barney's Farm as a mix between Menodicino Purps, Skunk, and Afghani. Grape Ape gets its name from its distinct grape smell. It is a pure indica strain that provides incredible feelings of relaxation that may ease chronic pain, stress, or anxiety.

Use For:

Stress, Pain, Insomnia, Depression

Effects:

Relaxed, Happy, Euphoric, Sleepy, Uplifted

Constituents:

15–23% THC

0.07% CBD

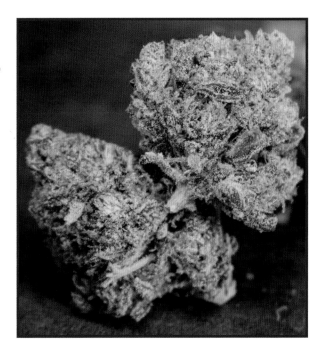

GSC (Hybrid)

Characteristics:

Formerly known as Girl Scout Cookies, GSC is the recipient of multiple Cannabis Cup awards and is a highly covetable hybrid strain. Its sweet yet earthy aroma profile and euphoric and relaxing effects make this strain very appealing for patients who need pain and stress relief.

Use For:

Insomnia, Stress, Depression, Lack of Appetite, Pain

Effects:

Happy, Relaxed, Euphoric, Creative

Constituents:

17–28% THC

0.09–0.2% CBD

0.4–2.2% CBG

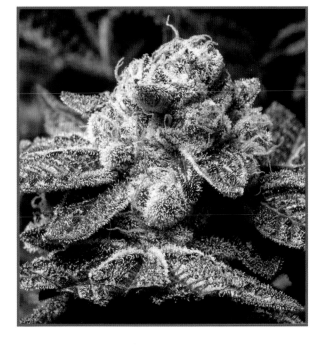

Harlequin (Sativa)

Characteristics:

A sativa-dominant strain that was produced from the genetics of Colombian Gold and Nepali indica, Harlequin is very well known for its very reliable production of CBD—usually with a ratio of five parts of CBD to every two parts of THC. This high CBD percentage gives Harlequin the ability to effective relieve symptoms of pain and anxiety.

Use For:

Stress, Pain, Depression, Inflammation, Headaches

Effects:

Relaxed, Focused, Uplifted, Happy, Energetic

Constituents:

4–7% THC

8–16% CBD

0.2–0.9% CBG

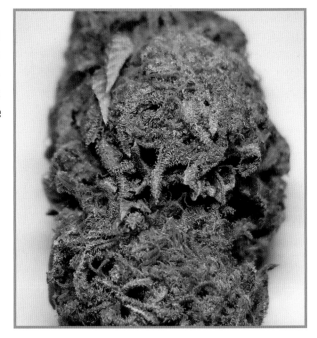

Headband (Hybrid)

Characteristics:

Headband is the progeny of the long-time cannabis favorites OG Kush and Sour Diesel. It has lemon-tinged scent with hints of Sour Diesel's gasoline-like smell. Its effects are long lasting but are know to come on slower than many other strains.

Use For:

Stress, Pain, Depression, Insomnia, Headaches

Effects:

Euphoric, Happy, Relaxed, Uplifted

Constituents:

20–27% THC

0.07–0.2% CBD

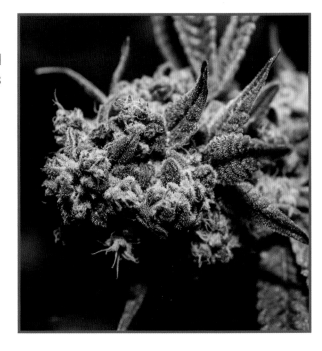

Laughing Buddha (Sativa)

Characteristics:

This 2003 *High Times* Cannabis Cup winner is a cross between Thai and Jamaican sativa strains from Barney's Farm. As the name implies, this sweet and spicy smelling strain will leave you laughing in an upbeat and euphoric state.

Use For:

Stress, Depression, Fatigue, Lack of Appetite, Pain

Effects:

Happy, Euphoric, Uplifted, Energetic, Giggly

Constituents:

18–20% THC

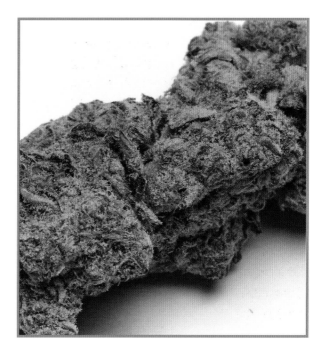

Lemon Haze (Sativa)

Characteristics:

Known and named for its very pungent lemon and citrus smell, Lemon Haze also has a yellow tint to its flowers from the amber colored hairs that grow on its trichomes.

Use For:

Stress, Depression, Pain, Headaches

Effects:

Happy, Uplifted, Relaxed, Euphoric, Energetic

Constituents:

15–20% THC
0.38% CBD

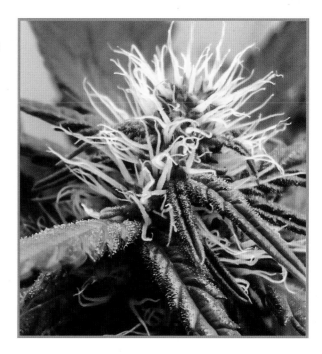

Lemon Jack (Sativa)

Characteristics:

The progeny of Jack Herer and Lemon Kush, Lemon Jack is a very potent sativa with heavy psychoactive effects. It is not as notorious as the strains making up its ancestry, but it is gaining a reputation quickly. Good for daytime use because it does not cause excessive tiredness, Lemon Jack can most definitely help those with anxiety.

Use For:

Stress, Lack of Appetite, Depression, Fatigue

Effects:

Energetic, Focused, Happy, Relaxed

Constituents:

Not Yet Measured

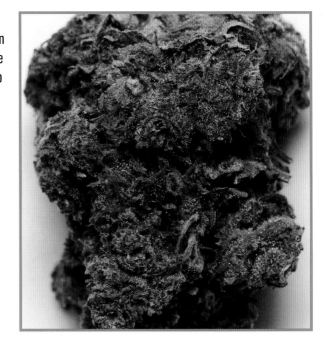

Lemon Kush (Hybrid)

Characteristics:

With a consensus agreeing that Lemon Kush is a blend of the Master Kush and Lemon Joy strains, there has been a recent surge of different varieties of the strain through breeders throughout the nation. Like its name suggests, it has strong lemon aromas with earthy undertones from its Kush progenitors. It creative and uplifting effects are perfect for soothing out the stress of your day.

Use For:

Stress, Depression, Pain, Insomnia, Lack of Appetite

Effects:

Relaxed, Uplifted, Happy, Euphoric, Energetic

Constituents:

15–26% THC
6.3% CBD

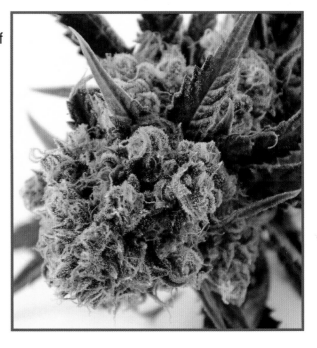

OG Kush (Hybrid)

Characteristics:

The genetic forerunners of OG Kush are still unknown despite its status as a seminal strain in west-coast cannabis circles. Developed in Florida in 1995 from propagators now known as Imperial Genetics, OG Kush has become the genetic foundation for many popular strains today. It smells of pine and lemon with umami undertones and is incredibly effective in dealing with stress.

Use For:

Stress, Depression, Pain, Insomnia, Lack of Appetite

Effects:

Relaxed, Sleepy, Happy, Euphoric

Constituents:

19–26% THC

0–0.3% CBD

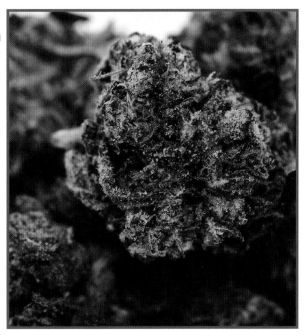

Presidential OG (Indica)

Characteristics:

A cross between Bubble Gum and OG Kush, Presidential OG has earthy flavors and lemon-pine aromas that are sure to overwhelm your senses. It has a fairly fast onset with heavy sedative effects.

Use For:

Insomnia, Stress, Pain, Lack of Appetite, Fatigue

Effects:

Sleepy, Relaxed, Happy, Euphoric

Constituents:

20–23% THC

0.3% CBD

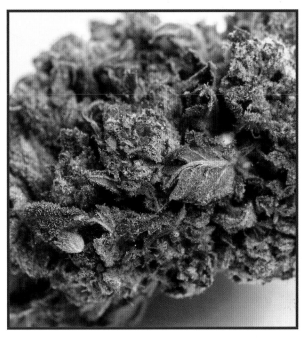

Purple Kush (Indica)

Characteristics:

This pure indica strain came from Oakland, California, as a cross between Hindu Kush and Purple Afghani. It has both relaxing and euphoric effects that are long lasting.

Use For:

Stress, Insomnia, Pain, Depression, Fatigue

Effects:

Relaxed, Happy, Euphoric, Sleepy, Hungry

Constituents:

17–22% THC

0.07–0.1% CBD

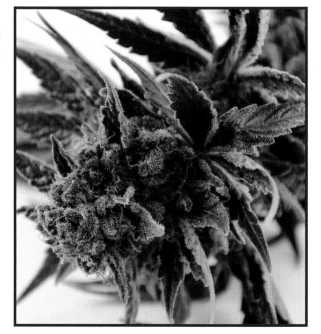

Purple Urkle (Indica)

Characteristics:

It is believed that Purple Urkle was first bred in California from a Mendocino Purps blend. It has a skunky and berry-like smell with a fast onset of effects that make it great for using before bed. It is very good to use for pain and relaxation.

Use For:

Pain, Insomnia, Stress, Depression, Muscle Spasms

Effects:

Relaxed, Sleepy, Euphoric, Happy, Hungry

Constituents:

16–26% THC

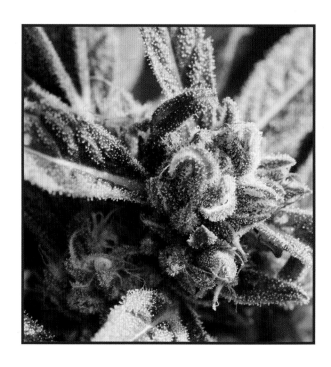

Strawberry Cough (Sativa)

Characteristics:

Known for its sweet smell and tendency to make even the most experienced smoker cough, Strawberry Cough is a potent sativa with a questionable history. It creates uplifting effects that are great for social situations. Very good for smoking during the day because it does not cause excessive tiredness.

Use For:

Anxiety, Stress, Depression Fatigue

Effects:

Happy, Uplifted, Energetic, Euphoric

Constituents:

22–26% THC

1% CBD

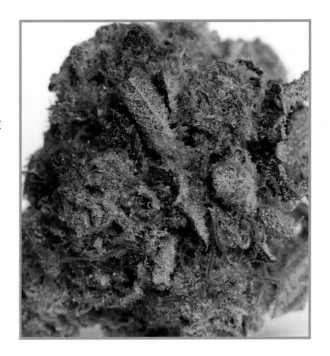

Sour Diesel (Sativa)

Characteristics:

Sour Diesel is a legendary sativa strain with a pungent, gasoline-like aroma. It is a fast acting herb that creates a dreamy and cerebral effect that can help with a variety of medical conditions. Sour Diesel first made its appearance on the scene in the 90s and is derived from Chemdawg 91 and Super Skunk strains.

Use For:

Stress, Depression, Pain, Fatigue, Headaches

Effects:

Happy, High Energy, Creative, Dreamy

Constituents:

19–25% THC

0.1–0.3% CBD

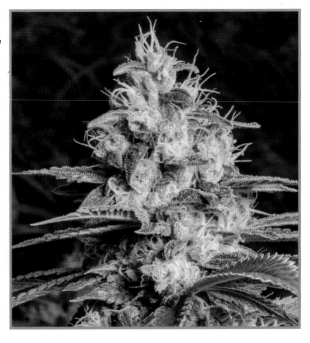

White Rhino (Hybrid)

Characteristics:

This very pungent and effective hybrid comes from a lineage of the White Widow hybrid strain and an unknown North American indica strain. It is a short and bushy strain that has incredibly high THC percentages and low CBD percentages. Flavor profiles cover an oaky and earthy profile, while its aromatic characteristics resemble sour berries. Highly recommended for medical use.

Use For:

Stress, Pain, Insomnia, Mood Disorders, and Migraines

Effects:

Relaxed, Euphoric, Sleepy, Happy, Uplifted

Constituents:

18–25% THC

1% CBD

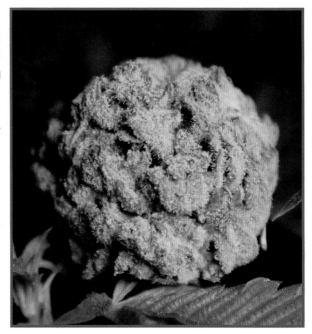

XJ-13 (Hybrid)

Characteristics:

An incredibly effective therapeutic and euphoric strain that is sativa dominant, XJ-13 is a cross between Jack Herer and G13 Haze. It can stimulate creativity and energy, but it will not produce a heavy feeling of paranoia, so it is great for users with less experience.

Use For:

Depression, Stress, Pain, Fatigue, Lack of Appetite

Effects:

Happy, Energetic, Relaxed, Creative

Constituents:

22% THC

1% CBD

1% CBN

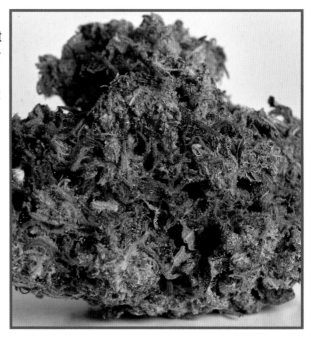